Praise for the *Voices of* Book Series

"Pure inspiration."

Shape Magazine

"...provides answers to practically anyone wondering 'What now?' ...this worthy collection succeeds very well."

Publishers Weekly

"Hearing others' stories is the most substantial aspect of any support group... It's the universality of the emotions that links these essays and puts the human face on what can be a very scary disease. For all patient health collections."

Library Journal

Other Books by The Healing Project

Voices of Alcoholism
Voices of Alzheimer's
Voices of Breast Cancer
Voices of Lung Cancer

Voices of Autism

The Healing Companion: Stories for Courage, Comfort and Strength

Edited by

The Healing Project

www.thehealingproject.org

"Voices Of" Series Book No. 5

LaChancepublishing

LACHANCE PUBLISHING • NEW YORK
www.lachancepublishing.com

Copyright © 2008 by LaChance Publishing LLC

ISBN 978-1-934184-05-9

Managing Editor
Victor Starsia

Editor
Richard Day Gore

Library of Congress Control Number: 2007943233

Publisher: LaChance Publishing LLC
               120 Bond Street
               Brooklyn, NY 11217
               www.lachancepublishing.com

Distributor: Independent Publishers Group
               814 North Franklin Street
               Chicago, IL 60610
               www.ipgbook.com

This book is available at special discounts for bulk purchases for sales promotions or premiums. Special editions, including personalized covers, excerpts of existing books, and corporate imprints, can be created in large quantities for special needs. For more information, write to LaChance Publishing, 120 Bond Street, New York, NY 11217 or email info@lachancepublishing.com.

Sometimes the journey from beginning to end is not always clear and straightforward. While work on *Voices Of* began just a short time ago, the seeds were planted long ago by beloved sources. This book is dedicated to Jennie, Larry and Denise, who in the face of all things good and bad gave courage and support in excess. But especially to Richard, who taught us by the way he lived his life that anything is possible given enough time, hard work and love.

Contents

Part I: Clouds on the Horizon

Part II: Caught in the Storm

Special Section

A Study in Hope:
A Mother, Her Son, and the Doctor Who Helped

Part III: Finding Shelter

Part IV: The Clouds Part

Foreword

The Power of the Storyteller
Aaron Liebowitz, MSW

In Native American culture, the power of the storyteller resides in the conferring of knowledge, which creates a connection between a community's past and its future generations. There is a special power that comes from the voice of someone who has a unique and life-defining experience and has the courage to share the experience with others. Such power is not only felt by the person who shares the experience but by those who listen. I have personal experience on both sides of this phenomenon, through my participation in two volumes of the "Voices Of" book series.

My first exposure occurred when I was asked to contribute a piece for the *Voices of Alzheimer's* volume following the death of my mother from that disease. I was a reluctant contributor at the time; initially, I did not feel comfortable writing an account of such a personal matter. In retrospect, I realized that the telling of my story, of my mother's story, of *our story*, was indeed part of the healing I needed.

Voices of Autism brings me back to the power of storytelling. This time, I do not speak from the perspective of being personally touched by this baffling disorder, but rather by the challenge of attempting to be part of the solution for the many who are touched by autism. As the director of a large agency that serves many children and adults on the autism spectrum, I am struck by the power of the testimonies contained in this volume. These accounts are from parents, relatives, friends and caregivers of children on the "spectrum," and the moving and inspiring words from individuals who themselves struggle to live with and understand their form of autism.

These stories are immediate and compelling. They call on me to be more aware in my thoughts, feelings and judgment. As I read each story, the stream of events, discoveries, feelings and challenges expand my appreciation and understanding of how this disorder has touched each contributor in a unique way. Yet, similar themes vividly connect each story to the next. From the shock of discovery to the piercing awareness of how autism manifests itself within a loved one, there is a palpable sense of shared experience—of community—to be found in these pages.

Moreover, these stories represent a unified voice, a powerful voice that calls out for us to make every effort to be in the moment with those individuals and families, and be there in the right way. For those of us who practice our professions in the disciplines of education, psychology, social work, psychiatry, neurology, speech pathology, occupational and physical therapy and others, *Voices of Autism* instructs us to listen not only from a base of knowledge, but also from our hearts. Each message presented here speaks of how all of us can be a catalyst for providing new focus and meaning to life.

Finally, it is hoped these stories will remind researchers who are seeking answers for the causes and cure for autism, that… "a child is waiting."

Aaron Liebowitz, MSW, is the Executive Director of Adults & Children With Learning & Developmental Disabilities, Inc., a leading not-for-profit agency founded in 1957 that proudly serves the needs of individuals with developmental disabilities and their families. The ACLD's mission is to provide the opportunity for children, teens, and adults with developmental disabilities to pursue enviable lives, increase their independence, and improve the quality of their lives. Located on Long Island, New York, ACLD employs over 1,000 staff members across more than 70 program sites in Nassau and Suffolk counties.

Foreword

The Power of Numbers

Denise D. Resnik

When you raise a child with autism, numbers become a major part of your life. Since our son, Matthew, was diagnosed more than a dozen years ago, we've employed 74 therapists. His bedroom closet is lined with 25 large, 4-inch, three-ring binders filled with single-spaced, typed progress reports documenting years of early intervention. In the category of chewed items, we have shirts: 132 in less than a year; remote controls: 14; and because of his fascination with unraveling and depositing entire rolls of toilet paper, overflowed toilets: 58 (this has earned us the "preferred customer status" at Roto-Rooter, which we now have on speed dial). Eyeglasses destroyed and repurchased: 17; school concerts performed: 3 (though he only sang at one); nights per week he ends up in our bed just wanting to cuddle: 3. Times he said "I love you" without being prompted: 0, although we know that he does.

What we have not tracked is the number of times we've cried or laughed, the times we have thrown up our hands in frustration or the times we've had to explain that our son has autism. And while Matthew has made tremendous progress, he remains seriously impacted by the disorder and, over the past 16 years, so have we.

Just after Matthew reached his first birthday, my husband Rob and I began to notice a change. He was withdrawing into a world of his own. We began searching for answers, but at the time there was little support and very few resources. One year later, Matthew received the diagnosis, and doctors told us, "Love him, accept him and plan to institutionalize him." Those words were devastating. We simply could not accept them, and we didn't.

The following stories of courage, comfort and strength have been written by individuals impacted by autism spectrum disorders (ASDs) and describe their many different journeys. They have been authored by family members who care for children with autism as well as from individuals on the spectrum.

In reading the stories found in *Voices of Autism*, what becomes clear is the heterogeneity and complexity of the disorder. There are no easy fixes; no "one-size-fits-all" or "cookbook" approaches; no room for dogma. But even without identifiable causes and with no known cure, there is still hope. Our kids can and do make progress. They can develop their potential, especially with intensive early intervention. And they can continue to make progress and advance at every age.

Approximately 1.5 million Americans are affected with some form of autism. Its incidence has increased tenfold over the past decade, across all racial, ethnic and socioeconomic groups. It is four times more likely to occur in boys than girls, and it knows no geographic bounds.

In every community throughout the country, toddlers are being diagnosed with autism and their families are wrestling with what to do about it. By becoming informed about the disorder, learning what's being done locally in your community, at your university or through national organizations such as Autism Speaks (www.autismspeaks.org), there are many ways you can become involved. Consider volunteering as an aide to a child or adult with autism; identifying positions within your place of employment that could be well-suited for an individual who does well with rep-etition, concrete thought processes and functions; becoming involved in advancing supportive public policy; supporting and watching out for our kids wherever you go.

We need to make sure healthcare providers recognize the red flags of autism so children and their families may benefit from early intervention and receive the proper support with proven therapies and effective educational and vocational programs.

We need to encourage private-sector businesses to get involved and employ our adult children. We need "typically developing children" (those not affected by autism) and adults to understand and accept those with special needs, and model appropriate behaviors, social interactions and work habits for them. We need to create a more tolerant community that accepts individuals with autism and related disorders, values their contribution and appre-ciates their abilities and, in many cases, their brilliance. We need a significant increase in research funding to match the growth in the prevalence of autism. And we need a plan for how we're going to care for our adult children when we, their parents, are no longer able to do so. According to a recent Harvard School of Public Health study, the lifelong care for an individual with autism is esti-mated to cost $3.2 million. Caring for all people with autism over their lifetimes costs an estimated $35 billion per year.

For our own son and family, we immediately sought treatments and resources. We found very few answers, but we did find many parents facing similar situations, and thus a support group was born. I quickly realized how widespread autism was and how frac-tured was the delivery of services and support. Families were left to find their own resources and select their own palette of inter-vention services. Hoping to change this, I co-founded the Southwest Autism Research & Resource Center (SARRC) (www.autismcenter.org) as a place where affected families could find answers, help and hope. Working alongside Raun Melmed,

M.D., a developmental pediatrician and co-founder of SARRC, we were determined to serve not only as a convening vehicle, but to provide answers to questions and to question the answers.

SARRC, a community-based nonprofit organization, has since grown from a virtual research and resource organization operating out of our respective homes and business offices to an organization with nearly 90 employees based in an 18,000-square-foot Campus for Exceptional Children in Phoenix. The nonprofit has provided well over 100,000 hours of service and training to children, family members, professionals and paraprofessionals in recent years. During that same period, annual program enrollment has averaged around 5,000 for our therapeutic, training and other programs and services. Our research agenda focuses on the underlying causes and potential treatments for autism.

Over the 16 years of Matthew's life, we have laughed and cried through the struggles and triumphs of his progress. Still, I know there is more to be done, not just for Matthew, but for the thousands of individuals living with autism today.

Denise D. Resnik is President of Denise Resnik & Associates, a Phoenix-based marketing and public relations agency. In 1997, following her son's diagnosis of autism, Denise co-founded and served as board chairman of the Southwest Autism Research & Resource Center (SARRC), which today is an internationally recognized nonprofit organization dedicated to autism research, education, and community outreach, www.autismcenter.org.

Introduction

The Changing Face of Autism
Lynda Geller, PhD

Not long ago, autism was a mystery. It was not until 1943 that autism was first described by Dr. Leo Kanner of Johns Hopkins Hospital. (Asperger syndrome, a related condition, was described by Hans Asperger of Austria in 1944, but his work was not translated into English until 1981.) Yet the most recent study by the Centers for Disease Control on the prevalence of the disorder found that between 2 and 6 of every 1,000 children has a form of autism, a rate higher than the rates of childhood hearing loss, vision impairment, and diabetes.

Considered a psychological abnormality for many years, autism was widely believed to be caused by poor parenting. However, the initiatives by the National Institute of Mental Health to promote the important discoveries in brain research made in the 1990's (known as the "Decade of the Brain") resulted in a growing awareness that autism is, in actuality, a difference in brain function. This awareness caused the medical and scientific communities to come to a better understanding of the condition and to develop appropriate treatments that have made real differences in the lives of those affected by it.

What Is Autism?

Autism is an outcome, rather than a specific disease. With the development of ever-more effective brain imaging tools, including *computerized tomography* (CT), *positron-emission tomography* (PET) and *magnetic resonance imaging* (MRI) technologies, major advances in the study and understanding of the structures and functions of the brain have been attained. Recent studies have shown that many major brain structures are implicated in autism, including the cerebellum, cerebral cortex, basil ganglia and brain stem. Some important research has indicated that a contributing cause of autism spectrum disorders may be abnormal brain development beginning in an infant's first months.

It is becoming clear that there are multiple causes for the disorder, which we are just beginning to understand. Autism is thought to be inherited, with many genes playing some role in its origin. The discoveries made about the condition in the last ten years will eventually help us to understand the causes of autism, and that understanding will ultimately help us to develop specific treatment and remedial programs for individuals with autism. In the meantime, we must use our best current knowledge to provide treatment and support to optimize the outcome and the quality of life for these individuals and their families.

Autism is considered to be a "spectrum" of disorders that includes classic autism, Asperger syndrome, and pervasive developmental disorder not otherwise specified (PDD-NOS). Other, much rarer related conditions include Rett Syndrome, which affects females almost exclusively, and Childhood Disintegrative Disorder, an extremely rare form of autism that causes a dramatic loss in verbal skills as well as severe physical complications. Autism is also sometimes associated with diseases such as Fragile X Syndrome, a disability caused by a damaged X chromosome, and Phenylketonuria, a genetically-based development deficiency. All individuals with an autism spectrum disorder (ASD) share characteristics of impaired reciprocal social interaction, impaired communication skills and restricted, repetitive and stereotyped patterns of behavior, interests, thoughts or activities. There is tremendous variation from individual to individual in the expression of these characteristics, in both severity and manifestation. Individuals on the autism spectrum may have quite compromised cognitive abilities or may have excellent intellectual and academic skills. They may have more or less severe impairments in social interaction, communication, and unusual patterns of behavior. In fact, part of the problem in determining the causes of autism lies in the fact that the condition is so variable.

The Diagnostic and Statistical Manual of Mental Disorders of the American Psychiatric Association lists the following criteria to be used in diagnosing autism:

(A) A total of six (or more) items from (1), (2) and (3), with at least two from (1) and one each from (2) and (3):

   1. Qualitative impairment in social interaction, as manifested by at least two of the following:

      (a) Marked impairments in the use of multiple nonverbal behaviors such as eye-to-eye gaze, facial expression, body posture, and gestures to regulate social interaction.

      (b) Failure to develop peer relationships appropriate to developmental level.

      (c) A lack of spontaneous seeking to share enjoyment, interests, or achievements with other people, (e.g., a lack of showing, bringing, or pointing out objects of interest to other people).

      (d) A lack of social or emotional reciprocity (for example, not actively participating in simple social play or games, preferring solitary activities, or involving others in activities only as tools or "mechanical" aids).

2. Qualitative impairments in communication, as manifested by at least one of the following:

   (a) A delay in, or total lack of, the development of spoken language (not accompanied by an attempt to compensate through alternative modes of communication such as gesture or mime).

   (b) In individuals with adequate speech, a marked impairment in the ability to initiate or sustain a conversation with others.

   (c) Stereotyped and repetitive use of language or idiosyncratic language.

   (d) Lack of varied, spontaneous make-believe play or social imitative play appropriate to the child's developmental level.

3. Restricted repetitive and stereotyped patterns of behavior, interests and activities, as manifested by at least one of the following:

   (a) An encompassing preoccupation with one or more stereotyped and restricted patterns of interest that is abnormal either in intensity or focus.

   (b) An apparently inflexible adherence to specific, non-functional routines or rituals.

   (c) Stereotyped and repetitive motor mannerisms (e.g., hand or finger flapping or twisting, or complex whole-body movements).

   (d) A persistent preoccupation with the parts of objects.

(B) Delays or abnormal functioning in at least one of the following areas, with onset prior to age 3 years: (1) social interaction, (2) language as used in social communication, or (3) symbolic or imaginative play.

(C) The disturbance is not better accounted for by Rett's Syndrome or Childhood Disintegrative Disorder.

Individuals with Asperger syndrome share these characteristics of social impairment and restricted interests, but typically have advanced rather than delayed language development (although their language may be unusual in a number of ways). Individuals with PDD-NOS share these characteristics but to a somewhat lesser degree than would be needed to receive a specific diagnosis of autism or Asperger syndrome.

Across the lifespan, individual manifestations of all the diagnostic characteristics change in response to learning. Some cognitively advanced individuals may establish scripts and routines that diminish the outward appearance of autism. Others may develop additional psychiatric conditions that complicate their presentation. For those whose autism is less severe, teachers and other professionals may fail to recognize the autistic aspects of behavior and address only other, unrelated issues. This often leads to treatment that is not specific to autism, which may result in a lack of social progress at critical junctures of the individual's development.

Because we now view the spectrum of autism conditions as brain-based, and because we know that learning and experience can affect brain development, we have come to understand the importance of early and intensive intervention in the lives of those diagnosed with ASDs. Early intervention programs around the country have had a significant and positive impact on the outcomes for thousands of affected children. By helping young, autistic children acquire social, communication, language and cognitive skills at an early age, we give them an opportunity to embed these skills into their ongoing developmental processes. We must be equally diligent in identifying children with Asperger syndrome and PDD-NOS and provide them with appropriate interventions as early as possible: children with ASD who are diagnosed early and receive appropriate intervention are much more likely to be able to participate in inclusive educational programs and have a greater potential to achieve an independent and successful adulthood.

Autism conditions are outcomes, and there are multiple pathways to these outcomes. For example, one of the hallmarks of the disorder is social difficulty, which may have varying causes. A child may have trouble because he cannot process what is happening around him socially, either visually or auditorily. The outcome of this brain difference, however, depends on personal experience. Because a child with ASD doesn't jump in and do the social things that children typically do, other children may start to distance themselves from him or may reject him, and, as a result, by the time he reaches the teen years he may have had very few social experiences. The longer this goes on the more isolated he becomes. Thus, what began as a brain difference becomes a social interaction deficit—the eventual outcome depends on the social experiences that a child is capable of, or that others allow him to have. If we could understand each child's particular brain differences and generate treatment and educational plans that really target specific deficits, we might be on our way to individualizing our approaches to remediating some of the important challenges children with autism face. Today, an interdisciplinary assessment by, among others, psychologists, special educators, neurologists and speech therapists helps us understand young children and their strengths and weaknesses. Neuropsychological testing helps us identify these differences in older and more able children. Eventually, we hope that some of our basic brain research will lead us to a better understanding of how the autism spectrum conditions develop and allow us to make more revolutionary interventions.

Challenges and Hope

Having a child with autism (or a disability of any kind) is a big adjustment for any family. It is particularly challenging for parents who, while mourning the loss of their own expectations for their child, feel that the "clock is ticking" on getting early treatment and that they must act aggressively to find effective services and treatment. Compounding these problems is the fact that many areas of the country do not have an adequate cadre of trained professionals to provide needed care. Equally problematic is the changing eligibility standards for services that families confront when moving from one intervention system to the next. Children who received intensive early intervention may find a preschool or elementary school unable to provide proper continuance of that care. When children move from elementary to middle school or middle school to high school, they may find that support services are less available.

For the individuals on the autism spectrum, the transition from school to adult life can also be very problematic if needed support is unavailable. Families whose children have received intensive services for years through the public school system may find it much more difficult to obtain services for the young adult. This dearth of services is particularly acute for individuals on the autism spectrum who present with higher intellectual and academic skills, yet are truly disabled in social functioning and independence skills. It is critical that our society make available for pre-school and school-age children, on an equal basis, the educational and therapeutic services that are so important for an optimal outcome and also provide support for those who continue to be in need beyond school age. Families of individuals with autism experience a significantly poorer quality of life than do those with typical children or those with children with other developmental disabilities because of the ongoing worry and concern over their child's life experiences and potential outcome, and the disruption in family life and community isolation that having a child, adolescent, or adult with autism can cause. Programs that provide support for the whole family are sorely needed.

The last decade has brought about an explosion of research and knowledge about autism. However, our understanding of appropriate treatment is still in its infancy and we are not communicating well-founded research results to educators and families effectively. Because every child with an autism condition is unique, it is critical that we develop more individualized treatments based on actual brain differences. The advent of the use of Applied Behavior Analysis was groundbreaking in its success with so many children. It continues to be one of the most researched approaches to educating children with autism. However, other approaches have been developed and are being studied. We must continue to progress in our understanding of which specific treatments are best for which children. In addition, we need to do much more work on how to successfully include children in mainstream education without sacrificing their need for specialized treatments.

Parents and educators must be wary when examining unproven treatments. For example, in a recent review of social skills interventions in schools, it was found that very few approaches being used today can demonstrate any real effectiveness. In investigating treatments, it is just as important to put aside those that are ineffective, or even harmful, as to find what is helpful. Too many families, desperate for help for their children, fall victim to unproven and often expensive treatments, some offered by well intentioned professionals, others by the unscrupulous. Developing evidence of the usefulness of all of the treatments that are emerging is critical to the outcomes for this generation of children with autism. The media is sometimes a tremendous help in bringing information to families and the public at large, but other times the scientific basis, or lack thereof, of the information is glossed over in favor of a sensational story. For example, it may make better copy to report that autism is an epidemic than to report that the rates of incidence are rather stable and that the increased numbers of children identified with autism are due primarily to improved diagnosis and the widening of the definition of autism to include a family of related conditions. Those in the media need to be real partners in the campaign to understand and treat autism by presenting evidence-based information and helping the public understand the legitimate issues autism presents, and by giving a face to autism that supports individuals and families.

In the meantime, our knowledge of autism continues to evolve, and parents need to keep themselves informed. Science and experience give us reason to believe that with time, awareness, and the collaborative work from many fields , we will see the day when autism spectrum disorders are more fully understood and all individuals on the spectrum will be able to lead productive, secure lives.

_____

Dr. Lynda Geller is the Clinical Director for New York University's Asperger Institute and is nationally known for her work helping children and families with Autism Spectrum Disorders. She frequently consults with school districts around the country on effective teaching programs for autistic individuals.

Dr. Geller received a Bachelor of Arts degree in psychology and a Masters degree in school psychology from the University of Illinois. She received a PhD from the University of Miami in counseling psychology. Prior to joining New York University, Dr. Geller served for 22 years on the faculties of the medical schools of Georgetown University and Stony Brook University where she specialized in the evaluation and treatment of individuals with ASD and related developmental disabilities. She has developed innovative intervention programs for these individuals and has educated physicians, psychologists, teachers and allied health care professionals in treating those with special needs. She served as the Executive Director of Asperger Foundation International from 2004 to 2006 and is currently a member of the Foundation's board of directors.

The Healing Project

Individuals diagnosed with life threatening or chronic, debilitating illness face countless physical, emotional, social, spiritual, and financial challenges during their treatment and throughout their lives. The support of family members, friends, and the community at large is essential to their successful recovery and their quality of life; access to accurate and current information about their illnesses enables patients and their caretakers to make informed decisions about treatment and post-treatment care. Founded in 2005 by Debra LaChance, *The Healing Project* is dedicated to promoting the health and well being of these individuals, developing resources to enhance their quality of life, and supporting the family members and friends who care for them. *The Healing Project* creates ways in which individuals can share their stories while providing access to current information about their illnesses, and strives to promote public understanding of the impact such illnesses have on the lives of those affected. For more information about *The Healing Project* and its programs, please visit our website at www.thehealingproject.org.

Send Us Your Story

Do you have a story to tell? LaChance Publishing and The Healing Project publish the stories written by people like you. Have you or those you know been touched by life threatening illness or chronic disease? Your story can give comfort, courage and strength to others who are going through what you have already faced.

Your story should be no less than 500 words and no more than 2,000 words. You can write about yourself or someone you know. Your story must inform, inspire or teach others. Tell the story of how you or someone you know faced adversity; what you learned that would be important for others to know; how dealing with the illness or disorder strengthened or clarified your relationships or inspired positive changes in your life.

The easiest way to submit your story is to visit the LaChance Publishing website at www.lachancepublishing.com. There you will find guidelines for submitting your story online, or you may write to us at submissions@lachancepublishing.com. We look forward to reading your story!

Acknowledgments

This book would not have been possible without the selfless dedication of many people giving freely of their valuable time and expertise. We'd particularly like to thank Theresa Russell, Alice Bergmann and Amy Shore for their unending efforts to reach out to the people and organizations making so many contributions to this book; Melissa Marr for her invaluable assistance, insights and opinions; to Aaron Liebowitz and Drs. Doreen Granpeesheh, Jonathan Tarbox, Richard J. Kessler and Lynda Geller for lending their extraordinary expertise; and to the many, many people who submitted their stories to us, for their courage, their generosity and their humanity.

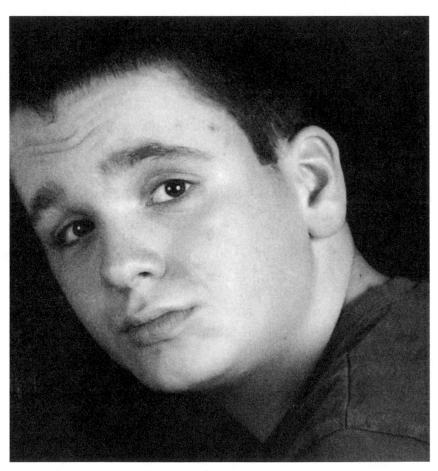

Michael Johnson

The Price of Talk
Michael Johnson

My name is Michael. I am 14, and I have autism. Some say that I am nonverbal, but I can communicate. I can say a few words that people who know me can understand, but I can't talk fluently. I do type with facilitation, but even that takes longer than I'd like. Not being able to talk is very frustrating. My mind knows what I want to say but my lips, tongue, and breath can't make it happen. Usually I try to say it but it doesn't come out in an intelligible way. Typing has helped me express my thoughts and emotions, and it has also allowed me to be appreciated as a person.

Typing is not a perfect substitute for talking, however, as it is not a usual part of conversation. I get upset wishing I could talk because I want to participate easily in conversations. By the time I type what I want to say, the conversation has moved forward. The time delay is unnatural. The only good aspect of typing is that I think before I say something, so I can be concise and can take into account how what I say affects others. People say that talk is cheap, but to me it has immense value. I wish I could afford it.

Michael Johnson is 14 years old and lives in University City, Missouri. He has been enrolled in the Giant Steps program for autistic children with inclusion in a regular classroom at his home school since prekindergarten. Now in the 8th grade, he excels in Latin, Algebra, and Communication Arts. Michael is apraxic and unable to speak. Despite fine motor limitations, he types to communicate with persistence and the help of word prediction software. Michael is thankful for the strong support of his parents, sister, and nanny.

Editor's note: Michael is also an accomplished poet and his work can be found throughout this book.

Part I
Clouds on the Horizon

A Boy with Autism Speaks

Michael Johnson

No one knows why
But I must try
To live my life with autism
Trapped inside a body that refuses
To follow the orders from my brain
Or form the words I long to say
I try to make friends
Even though I don't know all the rules
Or like to follow the ones
I think I understand
Autism looms
A nagging reminder of my limitations
Yet I see possibilities
Why me? has no relevance
What now? My next hurdle
Who cares? They are my salvation
Where am I going? As far as I dare imagine
With the trepidation I cannot escape
How do I get there? One day at a time
When will I arrive? Never soon enough
But I relish the chance to try

Anonymous Asperger's
Chris Lee Moore

Everyone feels left out and unwanted at some point; we all think we don't fit in or that we don't belong anywhere. But what if you felt like that for almost your entire life, and for the longest time you didn't know the reason?

From the moment I entered grade school, finding friends was never my concern. At lunchtime, I always tried to find the farthest spot away from everyone, and never really talked to anybody. Pleasing my teachers was more important to me than pleasing my classmates.

When I was disciplined for the first time, it was as if the world collapsed. Getting in trouble at school was unacceptable to me. I shut myself in my locker and then in a closet once I got home. From then on, I made a concerted effort to be the teacher's pet.

This only distanced me further from everybody else.

In the third grade, I was introduced to a much more sweeping form of discipline. If the class was acting up, everybody got punished. It didn't matter if I was sitting quietly trying to work; I'd be forced to sit inside at recess or write lines for things I didn't do with everyone else. These were the most humiliating experiences of my young life and I despised my fellow students for them. From then on I avoided everyone. I would head for the back of the play-ground by myself and not let anyone near me.

Things only got worse as I went from elementary to middle school. I kept away from the other students and disliked them more because I had to sit in with them in detention. They noticed my distance and teased me for it. I would hide to avoid them and I would often talk or sing to myself to keep myself company and keep the rest of the world out. In the fourth grade my parents packed us all up and left the Fort Worth home I'd always lived in and moved us to Arlington, just to keep me from going to a high school where they feared I'd be shot for being different.

One day, years later, my mother, an elementary school nurse, was told of a child who suffered from Asperger syndrome. She read about the symptoms–specifically, those of struggles in social inter-action and unusual language skills–and suddenly realized that I had this condition.

I was already nineteen.

In some ways, I don't think I've ever completely understood this condition and I'm not sure I've ever really wanted to. I went to a counselor who specialized in this disorder, but not for very long. How can you truly understand something you've had for more than half your life without knowing it is a disorder?

By this time, I wasn't spending all of my time alone anymore. I had spent the past few years attending a theater school. I found that when I could get on a stage and become another person, I could free myself of all my inhibitions. I'd always felt like I could be a performer, and now not only did I have a place in which to do it, I was among others like me. Maybe they weren't autistic, but at least they shared some of my interests. For the first time in forever, I found someplace where I truly fit in.

More fitting in soon followed. In college, I became the school's biggest sports fan, and gained praise from the athletes and coaches for it. They gave me shirts and even rides on the team bus. I found an interest in writing that led me to the student newspaper. Again, I found a group of people with whom I shared common interests in a place I enjoyed going to.

Of the many who deal with autism, I was one who had to deal with it unknowingly for a long time. Would the first years of my life have been less difficult had I known about it from the start? Who knows? Maybe not knowing there was a reason for my social inactivity ultimately forced me to find people who could truly be my friends.

I do know this. Today I look in the mirror and like who I see. Autism or not, I know I am different from everyone else.

And I'm not just comfortable with it—I'm proud of it.

Chris Lee Moore is a graduate of the University of Texas at Arlington and a former student at the Creative Arts & Theater School. He lives in the Dallas–Fort Worth area where he works as a freelance writer, sings karaoke, follows sports, and dreams of becoming a published author.

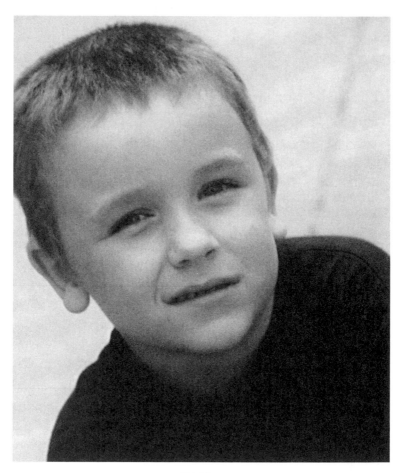

Al Trigg

Life with Al and Autism

Jason Trigg

When Al was born, everything about him seemed normal: he had ten fingers, ten toes, and his lungs and waterworks kicked in as soon as he was out of the womb. Al's first few years went by much as every other child's. He got yearly checkups, which always went fine, and he began jabbering around the age of two.

But Al's speech didn't seem to improve as time went on, at least at what would be considered a normal rate. Adults would try to get him to repeat words, but Al showed little or no interest. Since we lived in a small town that didn't afford Al many playmates, we assumed that not having other kids with whom to communicate was the cause of the delay. When he turned three, people began wondering if he would ever talk. I insisted he was just going to be a late talker and that everything would turn out fine. But eventually I yielded to pressure from other family members and took Al to the doctor for a few tests.

The tests started out simple enough—a physical exam for Al and a few questions for me. How did Al act at home? Was there a lot of stress in Al's life? The doctor said that everything seemed fine, and that Al had all the skills a boy his age should have. Like me, he said that Al would probably just grow into talking.

But over the next two years, I ended up having to do what no parent wants to do: run his or her child through a barrage of tests that were physically and emotionally exhausting for both him and me. When Al's social skills didn't improve, and even seemed to regress, the doctor recommended an electroencephalogram. I had never seen an EEG performed before, and it was heart-wrenching, watching my three-year-old son be put to sleep with electrodes attached to his scalp. All I could do was watch him on the monitor and wonder what I had done wrong as a father. The EEG came back fine.

As time went on and Al still wouldn't speak, people started to comment that something must be wrong with him. I stuck to my guns, insisting that he just didn't want to talk yet, but inside I was growing very concerned.

I was divorced then and had just started a new job. Luckily, I located a center that was open until eleven at night, so it was perfect: I could work and bring home money to support us, and Al would be around other children his age, and perhaps he would start talking. But not long after he started there, the staff began to report odd behavior, such as trying to run off, biting the teachers and hitting other students. Eventually they decided Al could not stay there. It broke my heart; I had hoped that he might make some progress and gain some acceptance there. There was no other day care available in my area, and it would be a long few months until Al was old enough for preschool.

When that time came, Al needed another physical exam. We had new insurance and this meant a new pediatrician. This was the doctor who changed our lives. After the usual examination, the doctor asked if Al had a lot of stress in his life. I explained the divorce, our new house and the failed day care. Finally the doctor asked a question that almost floored me: Had Al been tested for autism?

He referred me to a neurologist, and an hour-and-a-half car ride later, Al and I were sitting in a doctor's office that looked more like a playroom than a medical facility. The decor set Al at ease almost immediately. The doctor came in, introduced himself to us, and then asked Al questions and had him do several simple tasks. He asked me about Al's behavior around the house, about how much I knew of autism and if I thought it possible that Al had it. I hesitantly agreed that it was a possibility. The doctor made a few notes and scheduled another appointment for us to see him. A few weeks later we met again, and he confirmed that he did believe Al had autism. He gave me information on groups, websites and various other places where I would be able to find out more about the disorder. As terrible as it was to hear such a diagnosis about my son, I left that doctor's office with the first sense of hope: at last we had *an answer*.

Since finding out Al had autism, I have discovered within myself a new understanding and patience. When I explain Al's autism to others, they seem a lot less judgmental of his sometimes odd behavior. I have since remarried and now Al has a mommy whom he loves dearly, and she feels the same for him. Aided by our knowledge of autism, Al's life is continuing to improve. His speech, while still lagging, is getting better day by day. He doesn't have as many tantrums. I attribute a large part of his improvement to the fact that we are better prepared to help him: we understand now that he needs some time to unwind after a sensory overload. We understand that his brain works in its own way and we have adapted to help him any way we can.

Now I know why the symbol for autism is a puzzle piece: with Al, after years of searching and searching, the piece is in place. We got our answer, and it's allowed us to get on with our lives and the business of giving Al the care he needs and deserves.

Jason Trigg resides in Illinois with his wife and seven-year-old son, Albert.

What Is

Kimberly K. Farrar

"Can you feed the doll?" the therapist asked. When our daughter didn't react, the therapist pulled out a bottle of soap bubbles and started blowing. Laura, our daughter, was busily running her fingers back and forth across a green rubber doorstop as the bubbles, unnoticed, lazily drifted to the floor around her. My husband Jeff and I looked on while the therapist scratched notes onto the forms on her clipboard. She did not view our toddler as we did, complete and affectionate; she saw symptoms and categories, deficits and pluses, checks in a row of small boxes. After many more evaluations, Laura was diagnosed with a pervasive developmental disorder (PDD), a name sometimes used to describe autism spectrum disorders.

When Laura was about a one and a half, my friend Jill came to visit with her daughter, Emma. Emma immediately marched over to my aquarium, pointed to the tank and declared, "Fish." There was something in the determination of her action, her attempt to communicate, that made me turn to Jill and say, "Laura doesn't point." I later learned that pointing is extremely important; the gesture demonstrates a connection with one's surroundings, a desire to both show and confirm one's understanding of the world. Laura didn't point, ever, so I began to sit with her to try and teach her the gesture. I thought maybe she just needed a little practice.

Laura reached certain milestones far ahead of her peers. Before she was two, she could recognize and recite the entire alphabet, count to ten, and name the colors. But still she could not say her name. I believed that she was just growing in a different way. Later, we learned that these extreme abilities are called "splinter skills." I imagined a graph of Laura's knowledge base as a zigzag of steep peaks and plunging valleys like the cardiogram of a heart attack victim.

She would sit for hours looking at her books and her father and I would proudly nod, thinking *how intelligent*. She would spin the wheels on a toy for twenty minutes and we thought, *she is so intense*. She would pick tiny hairs or dirt particles from the rug and examine them and we would think, *how observant*. So many of Laura's quirks, things that we cherished as unique to her, turned out to be symptoms of her miswired neurology rather than characteristics of her individuality.

At bedtime, she would babble incessantly in a strange gibberish. It was not the typical babble of babies that suddenly morphs into speech. I could recognize the exact melodies and intonations of fragments of songs or snippets of dialogue from her videos. But it was as if her brain was imprinted with language sounds, but she seemed not to understand that words have a beginning and an end; everything ran together in a jumble. At first, it infuriated me when I would listen to her download her scrambled messages instead of sleeping. Eventually, I realized that she wasn't misbehaving and that she had no control over what was happening to her. I began to lie down next to her and talk softly, trying to calm her, to stay with her in her tangled world as she unraveled into sleep. It would sometimes take hours. When I told people that I stayed in her room until she was asleep, they'd tsk-tsk me for spoiling her. "Just let her cry," they'd say. "She's almost two and a half now. You shouldn't be in there." But I knew she was afraid and I stayed.

She started having intense tantrums that didn't follow the usual wave of a child's fit. Most tantrums seem to have a trigger, gather momentum, crescendo, and eventually subside, but Laura's would quickly build to a high-pitched frenzy and stay there for an hour, maybe two. Other mothers in the park would try to commiserate: "Oh the 'terrible twos,'" they would say. I began to feel that I was a complete failure as a mother. Sure, their kids cried or yelled, but they could be managed. There was always some reason for their children's fits, but for Laura there seemed to be no cause and effect relationship, no pattern which I could grab ahold of. Jeff and I ended up editing our actions that seemed to trigger the tantrums in an attempt to keep our sanity: don't put on shoes near the couch; only put milk in the purple cup; never cross the street at 30th Avenue; don't ever open the door while she's looking.

When I took Laura for a routine checkup, there was a new doctor at the clinic, a soft-spoken man from India. Laura sat before him on the examination table, her feet dangling over the edge. When he spoke to her, she didn't respond. She was mesmerized by the pattern of the tile floor below the blur of her swinging feet. He wanted to know how the potty training was going. I rolled my eyes to indicate that it wasn't working. "She asks for the potty though, doesn't she?" he inquired. I explained that she didn't talk too much. I now understand that in asking these questions the doctor suspected a problem that would change my life forever. His eyes locked onto mine. In a weak voice I asked if I needed to be concerned. The doctor explained that girls are usually more verbal than boys, develop earlier, and that by this time she should be talking. He must have seen worry in my face because he tried to reassure me that it was probably nothing. Then he handed me a speech therapist's card and recommended that I call. After I left his office, my immediate reaction was anger. I cursed him on the way home. When I explained to Jeff what the doctor had suggested, I ranted about how the doctor didn't even know our daughter. Who did he think he was? But I made an appointment the next day to have Laura tested.

Thus began the long journey of getting our daughter "evaluated." This is a word that I loathed because *value* is embedded in it: someone was determining the worth of our child's abilities. I had to watch her sit in the various doctors' offices, unable to point to the cow in the picture or answer the question, "What's your name?" She couldn't stack the blocks or roll the ball. She usually ended up hysterical because she didn't understand what was happening. I wanted to say, "Look. Look at her sweet face. Why don't you love her?" Why were these strangers important? Why were we going to all of these offices filled with toy-boxes and brightly colored chairs? We began to lose the rosy lens through which most parents view their children. I suddenly felt that I had to get to know Laura on new terms, terms of limitation and difference.

After that first evaluation, we tried to find a miracle toy: Jeff and I thought we just hadn't found the one thing that would crack open the shell that seemed to have closed around Laura. Jeff went out and bought a big pink and white dollhouse and set it up in the middle of the living room. Her playing with dolls had taken on new significance to us, since it was one of the boxes checked "No" on her evaluation forms. Laura was curious about the house and walked around it like a cat investigating a new chair. Our hopes sank when she picked up the mommy doll and began tapping it against the roof.

Hoping to prove to ourselves that Laura was simply stubborn or just didn't test well, we kept demanding, "What's this? What's that? Look at me," until she rolled over on the floor and started crying. Finally, after pushing her to do things that she simply could not do, Jeff and I broke down. We mourned. One day he would cry and I would comfort him, the next day I would cry and he would comfort me. Sometimes we both sat silently watching our beautiful daughter at the windowsill as she stared out at the trees. My heart literally hurt; I could feel it ache beneath my sternum.

We fought the idea of special education and the label it would forever place on our little girl, but eventually it became apparent that we had to put our pride aside. She was seriously delayed in all areas. We had to get her help, fast.

I quit my job teaching during the day and picked up some night work so I could devote my time to finding help for Laura. Even with my days free, it took three months to find and enroll her in an appropriate program. What had begun as a meeting with a speech therapist soon grew into appointments with a neurologist, psychologist, behaviorist, and audiologist. We had to meet with a city social worker and various school officials. Finally, after many school tours and conferences, we discovered a small school in a quiet neighborhood that felt right for Laura.

For the past six months, she's had speech therapy, physical therapy, and occupational therapy as part of her program at this school. The therapists and teachers use a lot of gentle physical prompting to guide her through her daily routines. The speech therapist skillfully teases out bits of language from Laura during their focused play sessions. It is language that has proven to be the most difficult aspect of her delays.

Now, I hardly ever lose her to that hypnotic world of pattern or motion, but it still happens. When I watch other parents talk with their toddlers, I am filled with a sense of longing.

Every weekday morning, I put Laura's pink Barbie backpack on her shoulders, kiss the top of her head, and shuffle her onto the mini-bus. When she gazes down at me through the big, square window as I wave goodbye, I am proud. We no longer constantly check Laura's progress against the developmental charts with their norms and averages. Laura is outside of the black lines that arc across the graphs. She makes progress in her own way, at her own pace. I am happy when she looks me in the eye and says, "Ma Ma" or "Want beans." The words come slowly. In the meantime, I shed my preconceptions of what is normal and try to look clearly at what *is.*

Kimberly K. Farrar is a mother, writer, and teacher currently living in Astoria, New York. She holds a Bachelor of Arts degree in creative writing from the University of Arizona, a master's degree in Teaching English to Speakers of Other Languages from Hunter College and teaches English as a Second Language.

Bunches and Bunches

Fred Marmorstein

The power of a child's love exceeds the limitations of autism. The challenge is in learning how to embrace those limitations. My challenge began when I saw my nephew at Christmas time. Josh was 16 months old.

"Hi, buddy," I greeted him when I first walked in to my brother-in-law Ron's house. Josh said nothing. "Santa will be here tonight. Aren't you excited?"

I quickly looked at Ron and wished him Merry Christmas. Ron smiled, picked up Josh, and exclaimed, "I love you bunches and bunches."

Throughout the holiday Josh cried, ran in circles, and hardly spoke. When he did speak, his voice lacked any emotion. He flapped his arms and banged his head on the walls. He repeated the same words. He couldn't even feed himself.

Ron kept repeating words, too: he kept telling Josh how he loved him "bunches and bunches."

It was a different story with me: I wanted to spank him. Surely they could see that Josh needed something. Discipline? Fewer toys? I knew there was something wrong, but I wasn't going to say anything. I just wanted to go home.

At the airport I looked at my own daughter laughing and playing. My wife and I were blessed with a "normal" daughter. I never said that word because it would have sounded offensive, but I was secretly grateful that I didn't have to deal with Josh.

Josh's problems prompted Ron and his wife Julie to take action. Ron called me one night and told me he thought Josh had autism.

"What does that mean?" I asked ignorantly. I pictured a kid rocking alone in a corner, holding onto his knees, slobbering, unable to communicate.

"It means Julie and I have a lot of work to do."

"I noticed something strange about him when we visited you guys last Christmas. The way you kept repeating things to him." I waited for a response. "Ron? You still there?"

Finally, he answered with a question. "Don't you tell Elana how much you love her?"

"Of course I do," I said.

"You shouldn't have to defend yourself for loving your child."

The words hit home and I thought a lot about them. I'd thought it was much harder to love Josh than to love Elana. But would I love my daughter any less if she were autistic? And if she were autistic, would there somehow be less to love? Of course not. A parent's love is a parent's love.

The following Christmas, we saw that a year hadn't changed Josh, but it had changed the people around him. I was more patient; my daughter was too. She held his hand and played catch with him. Julie spoke to him, giving him directions, repeating herself over and over until Josh started to listen.

And I started listening, too. I listened to Ron ask his son for a kiss. I listened to my own voice asking my father to tell me he loved me before I brought him to the nursing home that afternoon. And before I left to go home that day, I hugged Josh goodbye even though he screamed the whole time. I didn't care.

I've seen Josh many times since that Christmas, when I thought something was "wrong" with him. I've pushed him on the swings, splashed him in the pool, helped him cut his food, and talked to him about the pictures he drew. He kisses his dad and laughs.

Someday I will tell Josh how he helped me recognize my inability to love someone I did not understand. And I will tell him that I love him bunches and bunches.

The author is a former high school English teacher who now works as a freelance writer. Besides writing, he enjoys reading and hiking with his wife and 10-year-old daughter. He and his family live in northern Virginia.

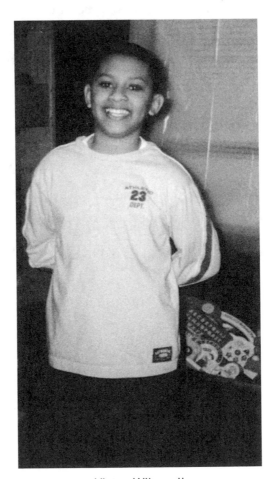

Victor Wilson II

Something Special
Linda Joann Wilson

"Go to sleep, little boy." It was after midnight and I was beyond exhausted. My eyelids were heavy and all I wanted was rest. His soft hums filled the room. A few minutes passed and the humming grew louder. "Hmmmmmm." He jumped from his bed and ran into mine, where he still hummed, as if neither bed gave him comfort. I had resolved to make him sleep in his own bed, where I once again placed him.

"Stop that!" Across from us, my five-year-old daughter slept soundly in her toddler bed. My little boy did not stop humming. I became enraged and whacked him. "Go to sleep!" I yelled. He still hummed as if he hadn't been reprimanded. *Something is wrong with this child*, my inner voice said. *No, he's fine, he wants to frustrate me but I will not let him.* "Hum yourself to sleep all you want. I'm going to bed!" I trudged back to my bedroom. One o'clock in the morning and still I heard the sound he pushed through his pressed lips. At three, I surrendered to darkness and permitted the irritating hum to lull me into a fitful sleep.

You should have him checked out, maybe something is wrong. It's the first thought I had as I awakened. My husband had said the same to me, right before I drifted off. Twice before, I had been advised to have him tested, once by my sister and once by a friend. *You can jump in the lake and take your advice with you. There is nothing wrong with my son.* He just didn't like people yet. Living on Planet Earth takes some time getting used to. My son flapped his little hands, made grunting sounds, spun around in dizzying circles and gazed at the lights on ceiling fans. He used to talk but now he didn't speak in any form of English. Perhaps he mastered some foreign language while still in my womb. I used to watch a lot of subtitled movies during my pregnancy. Experts say babies can hear inside the womb.

Or maybe he's going to be a movie star and he's saving his real talent for Hollywood. See how handsome he is? Look at those big, beautiful, brown doe eyes and long eyelashes. His dark curly hair is finely textured and so soft to the touch. Who wouldn't want a good-looking kid like this to star in their movie? And you say there's something wrong with him. Girl, please! Look at your little rug rat running around everywhere, talking to strangers and breaking stuff. Your kid also has a very smart mouth. At least my son stays close to me and respects the property and space of others. There's nothing wrong with my son.

What do you mean he just bumped his head real hard and didn't cry? He's got a strong skeleton protecting his brain. That's why he didn't shed a tear. He's going to be a boxer with a strong chin, too. You'll see.

In the back of my mind there was worry. I'd made myself believe my own excuses. A huge lump rose on top of my son's head. He hadn't made a peep. Not a whimper. No watery eyes. Nothing! I cried for him. For us.

During a trip to the mall with my sister, my son repeatedly placed his fingers in his ears and winced at the sound of passing cars or the voices of people. "Why does he always plug his ears up like that?" my sister asked. "That's not normal."

I responded, "What do you mean it's not normal? Don't you cover your ears when you hear loud noises too? There's nothing wrong with him. Maybe there's something wrong with you. He has sensitive ears, that's all. Maybe when he grows up he'll be a conductor for an orchestra. Everyone has a talent. I just need to zero in on his and expand it so his real personality can emerge."

Six more months went by and still no change. My son watched while I played with his sister. He held on to a fork and waved it in front of his face, making the utensil become a silver blur before his eyes. Maybe he was going to be a chef, I decided with excitement, own his own four-star restaurant. His eyes clearly showed disinterest as I observed him. That humming went on and on just like a beat. I focused on his sister and started reading to her. He came over, took the book out of my hand and turned the page. I assumed he wanted me to read to him also, but then he turned the page, then turned to the next page and so on and so on. I looked into his eyes and finally a bulb illuminated in my mind. My hopes of him being a famous author were dashed to pieces.

He was not really there with me. His eyes were staring off into a world I could not know. Maybe galaxies far away from me, his sister, his dad, everyone. My dream of my handsome boy as some Hollywood child prodigy disintegrated.

The doctor snapped her fingers. I jerked. "Miss, are you all right? Do you understand what PDD is? Pervasive Developmental Disorder. Here is a handout. Do you have any questions?"

Silent and filled with astonishment, I shook my head no. I felt anesthetized. In no real hurry to leave her office, I remained seated. My son stood on the edge of the chair and jumped onto the floor. I felt like doing the same, but from a tall bridge in San Francisco. I left there without a clue about my son's condition. All I knew was that I would receive a report in the mail. Well, yippee!

I went home and cried, bawled like a baby. It wasn't that I didn't believe in God, I just didn't cry to Him that day. I had shut down completely. I had no idea what the future held for my baby boy nor how people would receive him. My "mean mug" was already perfected for when we were out in public. As soon as my son hummed for more than thirty seconds, we were guaranteed a few stares, to which I would glare right back. I didn't care if it was human nature to stare at the peculiar, I would not allow it.

The report came a few weeks later, filled with medical jargon of no value to me whatsoever. I needed a second opinion. Maybe he was a slow learner. I took him to be evaluated by a group of school board professionals: an audiologist, a nurse, social worker, speech therapist, occupational therapist, and psychologist. He was unable to complete the hearing exam. Maybe he had hearing loss and needed to see a specialist. *So, that's why his behavior was so weird.* I breathed a sigh of relief. That could be easily fixed, I hoped. Visiting with the psychologist last, he pulled me to the side afterwards. I felt nervous energy surround me.

"Ma'am, your son is mildly autistic."

"Artistic. Oh, you mean he's going to be a famous painter." I smiled and nodded my head.

He smiled politely. "No, he's AU-tistic. It's a developmental disorder. There's no cure, but if you get early intervention by placing him in school now, it would help tremendously. Do you have any questions?"

"Yes," I said, as my eyes watered. "Why me?"

I said my son would be something special and he is. Seven years later, he is verbal. He does not always express himself in full sentences, but I don't have to struggle to communicate with him. He has progressed by leaps and bounds. He loves the Disney channel, the Internet, and Alicia Keys is his favorite musician. His four-year-old brother harasses him every single day; he has no choice but to socialize. As for the humming, he still does it, but not often. If I catch him in the act, he apologizes, "Sor-ree," he says and stops the noise.

After receiving my son's diagnosis, I had to stop the humming noise inside my own head. That droning sound of denial wouldn't allow me to see what was plainly visible. Unlike the bystanders who stared at my son's peculiar behavior, I chose to look away. It was much like plugging up one's ears to keep sound from penetrating. I had shut out reason.

I am most grateful that I did not destroy my son's road to progress by keeping blinders on. I've made peace with my heart and said good-bye to my dreams for my son. Now he can dream his own dreams and become whatever he is meant to be.

Linda Joann Wilson is a married mother of four and works as a government analyst. A Chicago native, she recently completed her first novel, *A Taste of Java*, and is working on her second, *Desperate*. Her short story credits include *Reappearing Acts for Crimes of Passion: The Anthology*.

Great Expectations
Michelle Alkon

When my younger son was 3, the doctors told us they thought he was going to die, slowly, after losing his speech, hearing, vision and muscle function. However, they also told us there was a test to verify their working diagnosis but that it would take seven weeks to get the final results. Seven weeks later, they told us that they were wrong and that our son had autism. My husband and I cheered, because we had just won the lottery: our beautiful son was not going to suffer and die. We learned a great deal about autism after that and after our older son was also diagnosed with an autism spectrum disorder. One thing we learned was not to allow ourselves to assume the worst about the prognoses for our children.

Parents of children with autism, or as we say, children "on the spectrum," do not get assurances. Instead of a clear path towards functional adulthood, we have a rocky, winding road with dead ends and cul de sacs along the way. In September of each school year, we do not get a target like other parents who hear, "By the end of the year, your child will have learned…" Instead, each year we hear a hope, that "we will keep working on this and try to see some improvement." We have learned to be realistic and optimistic at the same time. We celebrate each success as we persevere through each plateau. We focus on the process, the big picture and the long view, not on the end zone.

But we do not have diminished expectations for our children's future, and we do not focus on the disappointments. In this way, we can celebrate the small victories and look forward to many more. Our children constantly delight us, but they rarely surprise us with their abilities. When he was a freshman in high school, my older son, who has never been able to make a friend or have a playdate, was elected by his class to represent them on the student council (a highly prestigious job). They recognized his intelligence and his work ethic but also that he was one of them, despite his differences. When my younger son, who has sensory issues and significant autistic behaviors, turned 13, he celebrated the most beautiful and moving bar mitzvah (the Jewish coming of age) our synagogue has ever seen, reading directly from the Torah scroll and leading the whole congregation in song. If we had followed the path of diminished expectations, we would never have allowed our children to attempt these things. What a terrible loss for them and for us.

Parents of children on the spectrum are exposed all the time to what their children cannot do. At the same time, we honestly do not know what our children can do. It is a challenge for us to continue to hope and work in such a nebulous state. All we can do is stifle the doubts and take what comes as it comes. We support and we celebrate every success, whenever it happens.

Michelle Alkon is the parent and tireless advocate, coach, and cheerleader for her two children on the autism spectrum. She is an owner of The RBC Group, a research and consulting firm providing services to healthcare clients. She lives with her husband, Mark, in Newton, Massachusetts.

Part II
Caught in the Storm

Relief from Stress

Michael Johnson

Coming home by car
I stare out the window
and watch the world whiz by
It calms me
and helps just in time
so I can forget
the chaos of the day
Holding it together
takes a lot of work
when all I want to do
is give in to the monster
that forces me to be autistic
I hurry in from the car
switch on my video
and escape into a world
that is predictable and happy
Until I need
to hold it together again
when homework starts.

My Seat Rock

Kimberly Gerry-Tucker

"This is my seat rock," I said to the ants who soldiered across my knees. I gave each a careful flick, aiming for leaf litter and small saplings where I knew they'd be okay. They were resilient creatures with secret societies. But the rock was *my* real estate. In the castle of the woods, fifth grade was far behind me; with barely a neural pathway reserved to recall erasers, white sweaters with pearlized buttons and laughter like acid rain.

I didn't get diagnosed with the Asperger's until I was an adult, of course, but I already owned it. It was me. I was *it*. And that was alright. I didn't know what "it" was; I just knew I was different from the others. And I spent a lot of time on my seat rock.

My jiggly bottom and bruise-speckled thighs fit just right inside the natural rock chair, my legs dangling over the rock face; a good ten feet from the forest floor. Above me, I needed only to hoist myself up a few feet and I'd be standing on the top of the big rock where I could stretch out cat-like and pick mica all day; even the smoky black kind. I swung my legs and adjusted my elbows on rock armrests. Pin-dot sized red insects mesmerized me as they always did; gliding hypnotically over the rock terrain surrounding me. The alive speck-dots of blood-red color had adventurous missions to get on with; over the moss-stained crannies and sparkly pink quartz deposits.

I adjusted my tailbone into my rock furniture and let my legs and arms become limp things separate from me. My eyelids fell closed part way. Maple tree arms swayed high overhead; rustling their leaves in a swishing chorus. I tried to catch sight of the wind itself but it proved elusive. Even the isolated night creatures in the caves were glimpsed from time to time: a swift deer, a meandering skunk, an amber-tailed fox. But the wind remained invisible; a conductor to lulling leaf choruses, a cracker of dry hollow limbs. Tall solid trees creaked and scratched limbs together, singing. They leaned to and fro, dancing.

During the day the woods were not ominous; unless of course they were pillaged by "the others." I could see them, playing there on the cul de sac with their softball, metal bat and tanned limbs. Their insolent shouting invaded my music.

I tipped back my head; an intricate granny afghan of trees holding hands was my ceiling. Stitches of cloudless blue peeked around the silvery bellies of leaves in shades of green from pea and celery to emerald. A mosaic of sunlight played kaleidoscopic games with me. A feeling I could not name rose up from my chest, humbling me; it was almost too much to bear. I would surely cry.

I was startled by an inchworm dangling on an almost invisible silk, aiming to make purchase upon my unsuspecting nose. I gently pinched the gossamer lifeline between my hang-nailed forefinger and dirt-smudged thumb. Leaning foreword, I was able to relocate the little lime green body to a nearby branch. The silk reattached to the errant limb effortlessly.

I wanted to hug it all. My arms raised up, wincing at the gunshot bursts of laughter, and crack of the bat from "the others" in the road.

For a microsecond, the off-white planet was impossibly close to my vision. With a dull thunk it smashed into the bone below one eye. I couldn't process what the assault was at first, even when I saw it, with its dirt-encrusted half-moon seams rebounding off my seat rock.

My eyes widened to full moons as my fingers poked the stinging cheekbone for damage. I recoiled in surprise and wonder at this startling new sensation in my face; sat up straighter as I pressed at the tender swollen skin across my sore cheekbone.

Then came mounting sounds of invasion. *The others were coming!*

I hoisted up and out of my seat in the boulder's face—*blurs of the others, running the paths, hemming me in.* When I hit the earth, my legs crumpled and spilled me three feet down the incline; which was always the way.

Richard nearly crashed into me. "It went over here—*what the fu*—where did *you* come from?" he said.

I studied the indented place in the crooked pine's massive trunk where long ago someone had encircled it with wire which was now rusted and still clearly visible in places. The resilient tree had grown around it, bulging. Its encroached midsection, like the fat roll on a middle-aged man, had been trying to maintain its dignity for all the time since it had been crudely defaced. It grew upright, proud, though slightly bent, with long graceful pine arms.

Richard pushed past me, nearly tipping me down the path on my face but my elbow went out and knocked into the tree. I fell into it, and all-out hugged the crooked pine; *thanks for catching me.* "Where the fuck's my ball? You better not got it, Mutation," Richard said to me; making sure his baseball cap was on as tight as could be and smack dab center backwards. "Yo, Billy man? You see it in there? I know I saw it go past right where you're at!"

Billy was rooting in the prickers, gently lifting branches and peering into the tangle. My eyes surveyed the woods and noted an off-white contrast of color against the siennas of the leaves. I pointed.

It was four feet in front of my rock, half concealed by moist rotting leaves. With my eyes, I followed the route it must've taken, imagined it bumping along my tree-root steps to settle there off the path. Then I noticed her! *How had she gotten by me?*

Jen-nigh-fer was standing on top of my rock, walking its length, her hand cupped over her eyes to "better find" their errant projectile. Surely I *would* cry. She was treading all over the rarest black mica and on the quartz. I hated her denim top trimmed with fluffy pink balls. She had matching denim shorts, with yet more useless balls. If it were my outfit, I noted mentally, I would've chopped off the balls and put them in a plastic container with a lid. My parents supplied me, their only child, with all sorts of containers for just such collections.

"There it is!" Jen-nigh-fer squealed. Jen-nigh-fer pointed and Billy ran to the spot. Her parents called her Jennifer when it was time to call she and her brother in for meals. The others called her Jen. I called her nothing aloud, but in my mind I pronounced the middle syllable with a long 'I' sound because that made sense to me. She was Jen-nigh-fer; accent on 'nigh.'

I had been pointing the whole time and no one had noticed.

"I got it!" said Billy, beaming a yellow-toothed smile. He handed the ball over to Richard.

"Figures, my best ball..." he said, inspecting it. Richard wiped it on his polo shirt, striped like Charlie Brown's from the comic strip and whistled with two fingers in his mouth for all the others to get back to "the game."

I shrunk into the crooked pine.

Richard called, "Move your ass Jen! It was three to two. We were ahead. Move it!"

"Hey!" called Jen-nigh-fer. "I never noticed there was so much shiny stuff on this big rock. I quit!"

I reached for the squirt bottle that bulged in my big pocket. I'd been using it to mist my tongue and to make my rock change colors. I wanted to scream at Jen-nigh-fer, *'It's called mica, idiot!'* I wanted to nick off the tip of her pert nose with the handle of my bottle. Jen-nigh-fer sprawled out on her belly and commenced to pick long sheets of mica off the rock and put them in her pockets!

"She wants to play house with the scumbag!" I heard Billy call from whatever base he was occupying.

Jen-nigh-fer lifted her head and looked down till she was looking me square in the penetrating gaze.

"Oh my Gawd, Mutation! Your face is purple!" Jen-nigh-fer said.

My chest was heaving. I was aware of how form-fitting my sleeveless top was. It was one from the big garbage bag of things the kids of my mother's friend used to wear. Jen-nigh-fer was giving my body the "once-over." My face throbbed.

Jen-nigh-fer smoothed her shorts and hopped onto the path in front of me. She was a cheerleader like her mother before her. "Like, did the ball hit you?" Jen-nigh-fer asked, smiling.

In my mind, the water bottle whizzed through the air and came down again, removing a chunk of sun-kissed meat from her arm. Square on the arm that did the mica-picking. The candy apple color of the blood spurting from the gash made me smile. In my mind Jen-nigh-fer's mouth made a big 'O' and she screamed. The blood turned her pink balls red.

"Hey is anybody in there?" Jen-nigh-fer said. Waving her fingers in front of my face broke the dream-state and got me to running.

My mind did not differentiate between paths and bushes. It told me to get to my yellow house via the shortest means possible even if it meant straight through the pricker bushes.

My rubber-soled shoes slapped the pavement of my uphill drive-way at last; my thighs burning. *Something felt wrong in one of my sneakers.* My lungs could not keep up with my exertion. I could not catch my breath; I climbed the chipped concrete steps with a squishy left foot and stood on the porch.

My mother opened the door and greeted me full face. I saw her expression change from one of "hello there kid" to *"Jesus H. Christ!"*

A wide sheet of blood had cascaded down my leg from a five-inch gash in my thigh and pooled in my shoe. I was ushered past the rosy-cheeked paper Santa that was too jolly for my mother to take down from the living room wall. Things like that made her happy. Like the red garland still draped over the parakeet cage and the plastic Rudolph on the cellar door.

As she ran the bathwater for me, she was going on about some-thing but I was thinking of my mica vial; my Pixie dust. Later I would settle under my heavy blanket and shake the corked bottle of mica… Every time I did it was more powder-like; shimmery, magic. I would keep it by my side all night; perhaps it would ward off the night terrors that awakened me with silent screams caught in my throat.

Most baths were long affairs, and I often forgot to use soap. Sometimes the guttural sound of the toilet when I got nerve to press the handle down would send me running from the room and into a place in the house where the birds tweeted and my pet frogs swam in tanks. I would stand before the toilet lever a long time, afraid to push down the handle…

I took such silent baths that my mother called to me every ten minutes. "Are you all right in there? I don't hear you making a sound." I learned to make a splash in the water every now and again.

I lay in bed that night with my horror novel beside me. I had to do all kinds of things to make myself feel. Like our first winter in the yellow house when I would sneak out late at night and walk barefoot under the street lamp. It seemed I had to do all kinds of things since we moved from the beloved gray house—like walk barefoot in snow and read things that scared the hell out of me; just to feel. I ached for the old house and could not fill its absence. I cried for it at night alone and blamed the move for every terrible thing.

Kimberly Gerry-Tucker's short stories have appeared in *Women from Another Planet*, *Hearing Health*, *Planet Vermont Quarterly*, and *KALEIDOSCOPE*, to name a few. Her recent book, *Reborn Through Fire*, was ghostwritten for a burn survivor and will be available soon at www.survivorshope.org.

One of Those Parents
Carla Charter

I am one of those parents who insist on a meeting every year to explain my child's disabilities to a new set of teachers.

But please understand, I'm the one who sees the hurt in my child's eyes from an insensitive remark or catches their tears because someone in their world just doesn't get it.

And realize that what you're hearing at that meeting is only a small window into what I deal with every day.

Not for 1 hour, not for 6 hours, but 24 hours a day, 7 days a week.

I am one of those parents.

I'm easy to spot. The crazy woman in the back row at a kids' sporting event.

Not screaming because my child hit a home run or missed a catch

But instead cheering because he almost hit the ball or, blessings upon blessings,

even somehow got a bunt.

And once in a while I'm there in the stands just giving a little thanks

That at the very least he didn't get hit by the ball.

Understand that in some ways my children's disability take away small pieces of their childhood.

So I jump at every chance for my kids to be able to just be kids.

I am one of those parents

Who helps their kids with their homework.

But please understand it's not as simple as setting them up at the kitchen table

and letting them do it.

On the good days it's being there to heap on the praise and make sure they keep their momentum going.

And on the bad days it's pulling them through the homework.

Problem by problem,

Sentence by sentence,

And sometimes word by word.

Insisting night after night,

week after week,

that they keep at it until they get it.

Even if their disability is making them feel like they never will.

I am one of those parents

who gets excited over little things.

A good math paper,

Learning to write a story,

ride a bike,

tie a shoelace.

But please understand

I've been there when they couldn't do these things

And day after day I still insisted they keep trying

Because something deep inside told me they could.

I'm the one that does the eye exercises every night,

not hoping for perfect penmanship

but praying instead for at least legibility.

I've been there when an expert said if and when my child
accomplished a goal

Only to see that child soar above their expectations

On their sheer will power alone.

Please understand I am not complaining.

My life has been blessed a million times over by these children.

They have taught me more about faith, hope, determination,
laughter and miracles,

than I could ever hope to have learned on my own.

Yes, I am one of those parents

But please understand my children's disability has made me that
way.

Carla Charter is the mother of three wonderfully gifted spectrum children. She has been a freelance writer for seventeen years and is working
on her sixth e-book entitled, *One Mind*, and a children's novel,
Gerontius Cameron, Detective Extraodinaire. She is a journalist and a
columnist for the *Quabbin Valley Voice* and writefromhome.com. Her
essays have been published in *The Misadventures of Moms and Dads*.

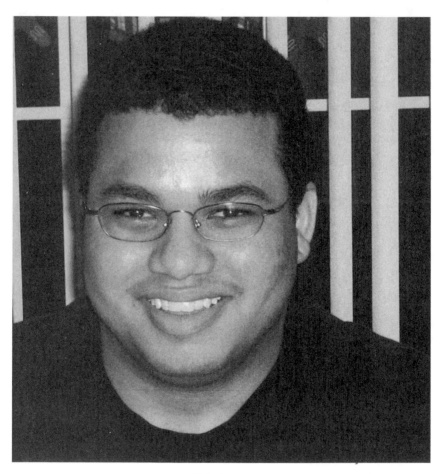

Kyle Luna

Postpartum Blues Plus Twenty

Claire Luna-Pinsker

Is it possible to have postpartum depression for over twenty years? I consider myself the first diagnosed case.

I adore my youngest son, my Christmas gift, a baby I begged my ex-husband for. Mothering him is draining me now that I'm older. For how much longer will I need to remind him (he's twenty now) to jump in the shower? It's a standard message I repeat over and over, otherwise he'll remain in pajamas. I long to do the same, which is why I realize I'm suffering an extended period of postpartum depression. My son has Asperger syndrome. Thankfully, he doesn't have a total non-communicative form of autism, but his disorder places a real strain on me as his main caregiver. My children are my heart and I'd gladly surrender my life for them, but there are times when I feel like I will be sucked dry by the relentless demands of an autistic child.

During my pregnancy, I realized he was going to be different. *In utero* he never rested, always twisting and turning, karate chopping painfully against my stomach. My abdomen stretched to an enormous size until, on Christmas Eve, he entered the world weighing in at ten pounds and six ounces. He nursed in a matter of seconds, constantly squirming, his roaming eyes taking in the entire world. My nickname for him was Panoramic Baby.

My Panoramic Baby wouldn't cuddle and complained if swaddled, preferring to lie alone on a blanket or catnap in a baby swing. In his toddler years, when disturbing symptoms intensified, I couldn't turn my back on him. Child protective devices were useless; he managed to maneuver his way around them like an escape artist.

Once I took him shopping with me, a harness zipped up his back because he wouldn't stay in a stroller. People gawked, but I felt he was safe, connected to me. While I looked through clothing, his strap safely secured around my wrist, he scurried underneath the rack. As I stepped after him, the leash went taut and almost broke my wrist. Following the leash, I found an empty harness zipped securely around a pole, and my son nowhere to be seen. He had escaped in a matter of seconds.

Panic-stricken, I screamed his name, rushing around, peering underneath other racks. *What kind of irresponsible mother am I*, I thought. Luckily, another mother found him (as he was about to get on the escalator) and took him to security. And there he sat, talking a mile a minute to a guard. His calm greeting was, "Hi Mommy." A con artist could learn something by observing my son's amazing capacity to outwit you.

When he was five I decided, after experiencing two frantic years of nursery school, that kindergarten was the answer to stimulate his mind and to harness his overactive brain energy. On the first day of school I wrote his teacher a note:

> *Dear Teacher,*
>
> *Here's my heaven-sent child. He's now in your expert hands. Please don't take your eyes off him for a second. He requires strict supervision and I do pay my school taxes! Please send my son home exhausted!*

As he grew older, new problems emerged. A big one was autistic rage. No one has figured out how to switch off autistic rage before it inevitably escalates. Once, I was rudely awakened at two in the morning by repetitive popping sounds, as if firecrackers were exploding in my house. The sound emanated from a broken speaker in his stereo system. I decided to calmly discuss the situation with him over lunch the next day, and requested that he disconnect the broken speaker because it was disturbing my sleep. Continuing to eat, he replied with a few grunts, his usual pattern of speech. When I asked for eye contact, an open bottle of ketchup whizzed past my ear, landing on the living room carpet, spraying the entire area. Then a container of fruit punch slammed against my kitchen wall. Before I could respond, kitchen chairs were knocked over as he stomped upstairs, kicking open his bedroom door, his foot splintering the wood panel. This was followed by a stream of cursing before his door slammed shut.

I was momentarily stunned by this outburst. I might have reacted by flying upstairs, kicking open his door, grabbing him by the neck and saying, "I brought you into this world and I'll take you out. Who do you think you are, destroying my home?" But this, of course, was an imagined reaction because I'm the mature individual who has to maintain complete control. Instead, hot flashes consumed me and, perspiring, I grabbed a bottle of carpet cleaner from a well-stocked cabinet. Struggling to the floor on arthritic knees, I scrubbed frantically at ketchup streaks. He sat in his room cooling down, with his popping surround sound system on full blast while I mentally planned placement in a group home, venting, unable to initiate this final step because I'm "Super Mom."

Later on, calmly apologizing for the millionth time, he robotically recited the correct way to manage rage, learned from attending a six-week anger management class. With a photographic memory he recalled exactly the appropriate words. As we scrubbed the walls together, he broke the tension by remarking dryly, "You can't even see where the ketchup landed."

People on the outside looking in might not be able to see humor in some of the dire situations my son's autism has caused; my sometimes warped sense of humor keeps me going. I once envisioned that my life would, eventually, be a total breeze and looked forward to being an empty nester, never imagining that I'd still be frantically trying to secure a babysitter for a two hundred pound twenty-year-old just to escape for a weekend. Over the years, my life has evolved to where I plan nothing without considering him first. I spend endless hours researching autism, reading everything I can get my hands on, continuing education on the latest developments. I speak to doctors, psychologists, psychiatrists, attend group therapies, and maintain direct contact with schools. Fortunately, his schools have been fantastic, willing to attempt anything to assist my challenged son. And he challenges them with his amazing wit, eagerness to learn and remarkable gift for soaking up knowledge.

During the past four years he's developed physically into a man, maturing to function in most classroom situations without supervision, using his own methods to overcome problems hindering him. If you notice him you'll see an adolescent suffering from acne, with a slightly awkward gait, kinetic eye movements and hand tremors. You probably wouldn't give him a second glance, but for him every day is a struggle to control the impulses his brain puts out. Literal in thought, with a wry sense of humor, his greatest personality trait is a strong sense of self-esteem. And no matter what happens, he's never depressed. In some ways it's a marvelous way to live, waking up and going to bed happy.

He's a young man attending community college for a degree in electronics, afterwards returning home and retreating into his bedroom. With no friends and no interest in making any, he's content to watch hours of television and be on his computer. His favorite phrase is, "I'm busy." He manages to write college-level essays, create elaborate websites and converse with friends in cyberspace.

To explain in detail, face to face, what he's doing is an impossible task for him. Emotionally and socially he's way behind his peers, still reacting childishly and impulsively, taking enough medication to sedate a horse. Thankfully, they ease some of his symptoms and they are taken willingly. Only once did I discover a collection of his medications, hidden underneath his pillow. An increase in his symptoms clued me in within a few days. His reasoning: "I think I'm better now. I don't need them." Self-medication permission was abruptly taken away.

There apparently isn't any medication for me, as my doctors repeatedly tell me, "You're doing such a great job handling him," or "Look how far you've come with him." Swirling in my long period of postpartum depression, I feel I've failed miserably. A pat on the back doesn't relieve my agony or erase his disorder. How can I let people know that at times I feel ashamed of him? Horribly, I've even thought about how life would have been if he hadn't been born. When he was initially diagnosed, little information about Asperger syndrome existed, and treatment programs weren't available. Today everyone seems to know of someone who has been diagnosed with some form of autism. Still, there's no cure and I can't place him into a cryogenic vault until a cure is discovered, though it's crossed my mind. Will I ever make the decision to place him in a group home that tolerates no defiant behavior? Could I live, realizing I gave my son away for a sense of normalcy? His disorder affected my marriage and is one reason for my divorce, but it also made me stronger. I've cried enough to fill several oceans: cried myself to sleep and cried from frustration. But I've laughed over his sometimes amusing antics and prayed for sanity to continue dealing with him.

I guess the prayers have been working. I continue slow steps forward, not knowing where they will lead or what's at the end of the road. Gritting my teeth and dealing with "postpartum depression plus twenty," I count love as my medication because I am my autistic son's caregiver and I love my son with super-mom strength, using my sense of humor as support.

Claire Luna-Pinsker is a retired pediatric nurse, wife, and the mother of three adult children, and now devotes herself full time to writing fiction, nonfiction, and essays on life. Her publishing credits include *Ebony Blood*, a romantic/horror novelette, *Newsday*, *What's Love*, *Affaire De Coeur*, *Our Journey*, *Manic Mom*, and *Born*; she has been published in *Romantic Hearts*, *True Story*, *Poor Katy's Kab*, and *Chicken Soup For The Caregiver's Soul*, among others.

Saturday Morning Imp
Kathryn Hutchinson

BAM. My bedroom door smacks the wall and I jolt awake, spying the figure outlined at the threshold. It must be 7 o'clock on the dot, for there stands Ramon, my Saturday morning imp. As he moves toward me in the dimness, I can just make out his toothy grin between boyish cheeks. Oh no. There in his hand is the dreaded white pen. I groan as…. "DEE, dee dee DEE dee dee dee DEE…" the "Michigan Fight Song" in all of its tinny, electronic splendor spilling from the pen assaults my ears. Ramon's cackle joins the din, and I reach out to grab him.

"You rascal!" I growl as he falls onto me in bear-hug greeting, howling with laughter.

Those darned researchers at the University of Michigan Autism Project sure know how to pick thank-you tokens their clients will enjoy. I could kill them at this moment. Didn't I hide that pen last weekend?

Ramon's ploy works, as usual. I haul my stiff body out of bed, pull on sweatpants, slip into flip-flops and follow his clomping down the stairs. Up since five, he has spent the last two hours as he does every Saturday morning, standing nose to the TV, shaking his musical pen or some other slim object as he obsessively watches the numbers advancing on the screen's digital counter, occasionally calling out "5:50!" or some other random time whenever the :59 turns to :00. I leave him with TiVo remote in hand and step into the kitchen, bee-lining to Mr. Coffee. Elmo's squeaky laugh causes me to cringe, and I brace myself for what's coming: "That's Elmo's Woooorld!!" How *does* that puppeteer hold that falsetto note so long? I guess I should-n't complain that *Sesame Street* is Ramon's latest nostalgic fixation, even if he is fifteen. It sure beats some of the other junk adolescent boys find fascinating, like the jagged-haired, tight-pants-clad bands of MTV or, worse yet, Adam Sandler movies.

As I reach up into the cabinet for a coffee filter, Ramon starts into his inevitable litany and joins me in the kitchen. "Mom, guess what show they did today? Number thirty-five eighteen, the one where Big Bird loses his teddy bear. They featured the letter M and the number twelve. And guess what tomorrow is?"

I grunt the necessary "Hm" so that he will not repeat the question, and dig the scoop into the coffee can, breathing in the rich Colombian aroma.

"Thirty-six thirty-three, the one where Rosita won't share her car with Elmo. It features the letter C and the number fourteen. Then on Monday..." and on he prattles, earnest, focused, and fast enough to rival a voiceover artist at the end of a new car ad.

I smile limply out the window above the sink into the gray driz-zle, ambivalent about the fact that Ramon won't be returning to his dad's till late afternoon. I glance at him every so often as I pour water into the pot and take down a mug, assuring him I'm listen-ing. "Mm-hmm... that's nice...."

I don't have the energy or the heart this morning to remind him, once again, that I, like most people, really don't care to hear all these endless and meaningless details he has stored in his brain, along with such odds and ends as the birthdays of everyone he's ever met and the complete layouts of two dozen grocery stores.

This boy could recite the alphabet backward at two and mastered his times tables through the twelves in one day. But at 7:10 on a Saturday morning, I must struggle to tolerate the stream of endless words. Three deep breaths later, I've mustered some patience.

I turn and rest my back against the counter to wait for the coffee and see him standing mid-kitchen, facing the TV with both arms bent upward, his left hand frantically shaking a long blue pencil. He is momentarily quiet, fixated on a familiar WTTW commercial. Bare-footed, his pajamas consist of forest green boxer briefs and a red Austin Powers T-shirt which blares, "Live and Let Shag, Baby!" in yellow block letters across his back. One idiosyncratic kid attracts another, I note ironically, thinking of Mike Myers with his oversized glasses, mutton-chops, and crazy snorting laugh.

Stepping up behind Ramon, I place my hands gently on his upper arms and lean in toward his ear. "Want some... pancakes?" I ask quietly.

He whirls around to face me. "Yes, Mom! Great idea!"

His joyous grin is infectious, and I am struck once again by the rawness of his emotion. He throws his arms around me for a ritualized bear hug, after which I am to hang out my tongue and pant, feigning breathlessness.

"Gotcha again, didn't I Mom!" he laughs.

"Whoa, you sure did," I gasp with an exaggerated groan.

I kiss his forehead, an act that no longer requires bending down, and he trots back toward the TV as the jungle-beat strains of the "Zaboomafoo" theme song fill the air: "The animals are friends of mine...." Still smiling, I turn back toward the cabinets and reach down to pull out the griddle.

Kathryn Hutchinson teaches English and is the Fine and Performing Arts Coordinator at a large high school in the Chicago suburbs. She holds degrees in English, women's studies, and literature, and is finishing a master's degree in written communication. She is the author of the essay *Leaving Literalville*, published in *A Cup of Comfort for Parents of Children with Autism*. Ramon is her only child.

When Tears Fall

D. "domynoe" Loeb

September 1996

Sullen and quiet, a remote island in a busy waterway, he lives outside the family that surrounds him. His silence is ominous, broken only by shrill screeching when his desires are denied or by the persistent drone of humming as he spins an object, any object, under his concentrated stare. Either sound continues for unending, unbroken hours. Then silence. He does not see the joy or care to join the dance of children as his sisters play merrily. Solitary, words unspoken, he wraps up within himself in a world of his own.

He is four years old. He is my son. My son... I don't feel it. Beyond a physical resemblance, no one would know it. An invisible wall keeps me from reaching him. Every effort is rejected, gentle loving touches ignored, kisses refused. Hugs become imprisonment—only sometimes, rarely, tolerated for mere seconds before arms and legs drop, back stiff as a board. His head turns away. My beautiful boy wants none of me.

A peaceful moment lost: my son is not in the house. We search, calling and calling, knowing there will be no answer. Finally found by his father a block away. A woman accuses this man she does not know of irresponsibility and neglect. Wild with excitement from his escape, my son evades all contact, climbs counters and tables, wreaking havoc on home and spirit. Once in his room, the screaming begins. A toy flies, crashing into the closed door. All I can feel is exhaustion and despair. There is no hope for me and my son.

My girls are nothing like this. They are bright and beautiful, sweet pictures of success. Articulate and well-behaved, though they still participate in the antics of any child. Normal. They demand my attention in a hundred little ways. Hugs, kisses, stories, gentle touches, immeasurable support. They even try to help with their brother. But too much and too quick for me, he's impossible for girls nine, seven and not quite three. His wall remains for us all, high, hard, impervious.

I stare at accusations: black ink on white paper with a blue letterhead. Nothing is wrong, they say. Yet my son is unsocial and unspeaking, quiet and still one moment, active the next. I see no end, no hope. Well-meant advice comes unbidden to my mind... since when have I needed advice? My girls are everything a mother could hope for. Empty reassurances, hospital letterhead notwithstanding, mean nothing. I have failed my son. My beautiful four-year-old boy is shut away from the world. Success crumbles to dust as tears fall, smearing a beautiful blue scripted name.

December 1996

Deep breath, grab his hand, try to distract him. It doesn't work. This place, my last hope, is too unfamiliar, too fascinating. He hasn't stopped moving since we arrived except for brief instances during the various evaluations. He lost control within half an hour of arriving. Racing down corridors to the next appraisal, sometimes responding to our calls. Usually his father chases him down. I get weary just watching him.

Between each evaluation there is a break. Now on our third wait. Until handed a clipboard of papers, his father stares at the television and chews on the pinky of his left hand. As always, I must cope with my son. Now his father fills out the forms, asking me the questions he can't answer. I answer most of the questionnaire. My son's father sees the kids long enough to take them to church and dump them in a Sunday school room, then bring them home when church is over. Being more involved wouldn't help him know more of the answers. My son is a stranger to both of us equally.

Finally called into the psychologist's office, I can barely pay attention as my son pursues his every fancy. First he wants the lamp, then the phone, both resting on the same table. A clock catches his eye and he attempts to climb the bookshelf on which it resides at the top. Denied, he picks up a toy to spin and goes back to the lamp table.

Then it hits me. The psychologist's voice becomes a blow to my heart and mind. Moderate mental retardation, developmentally delayed, and attention deficit hyperactivity disorder. I was right, there was something wrong. Bittersweet sorrow: I was wrong, it's not my fault. Bittersweet joy: in one moment, after months of struggle, I am freed, but now he's chained. Now there's hope and help. Tears fall in grief, dissolving guilt.

February 1997

Agonizing choices made. The class required for my associate of science degree in early childhood studies has been dropped. There are fresh wounds still, wounds reopened every time I went to participate in my internship: a preschool room with a dozen wriggly, wiggly, normal four-year-old boys. Constant reminders of what my son will never be. I can't see this every day, not yet. My relief has been overshadowed by my grief. My acceptance is so fragile.

One degree lost, but so much gained. There is peace between my child and me. The wall is dissolving. I understand him a little better. We're finally connecting. Peace is dawning between us. He still hums, spins, resists the play of his sisters, and has moments of stillness in constant motion. But he's beginning to babble and speaks a few words. Music to a mother's ears.

Home. Books and exhaustion weigh me down. I am greeted by humming as I open the door, but only for a moment. As the door closes, a little boy's voice, "Mommy! Mommy!" I climb the stairs, more cries of "Mommy!" from the girls. At the top, little boy arms wrap around my hips.

"Gi' me hug!" This is my son. I can feel it, no one could miss it.

"Hello, Kristav."

Tears flow, a healing balm over my heart.

Denyse "domynoe" Loeb has had work published in *COSMIC Speculative Fiction, Worlds of Wonder: A Webzine of Fantasy & SF, Lyrica: A Webzine of Romantic Fiction, Dragon, Knights, & Angels, Aoife's Kiss,* and *Beyond Centauri*. She graduated from California State University, San Bernardino, with honors and received a bachelor's degree in English with a concentration in creative writing. She currently lives in Georgia with her second husband, two of her four children, three cats, and a dog. She works as a writer and is the senior editor of Lilley Press, and manages Dreaming In Ink Writers Workshop.

My Life with Puddleglum
Rudy Simone

There is a character in the C.S. Lewis book series *The Chronicles of Narnia* called Puddleglum. At first, everyone thinks Puddleglum is as his name suggests—a wet blanket, a downer. But he is appointed a pivotal role in the story: he is the children's guide on their mission to save the land of Narnia. They learn to accept his dour manner and trust his judgment, and it saves their lives.

When I met Bill, my very first thought was, "He's good looking. Too bad he's so expressionless." I judged that he was not very intelligent; there was an absent look in his eyes. But when I got to know him over time (he was my landscaper), I realized that this was a charming, sensitive, smart man. I didn't know he has Asperger syndrome.

We began dating. If you know anything about Asperger's, you know that this was difficult, to say the least. People with Asperger's are often blunt and unromantic. Most cannot handle any emotional demonstrations, or what they see as someone making emotional demands upon them. Often they have a temper when stressed and can say hurtful things that they later might not remember. Communication can often be seen as a chore, as can showing affection, particularly in public. The list goes on and on. But I didn't know Bill had Asperger's at that time, because Bill didn't know it either.

There were many breakups, many the cold, empty, frustrated nights that I spent alone, trying to figure out what was making my sweet man behave so badly. I couldn't understand why he wanted to come over, only to sit there mutely and then fall asleep on my couch. I could not discern how an intelligent man could think that it was okay to call at 8 P.M. and say "I'm coming over," and then stop at five places on the way and not arrive till nearly midnight, when he only lived half an hour away. I couldn't comprehend how he could remain unmoved when faced with a river of tears and heartfelt pleading to be heard.

Then I found out he had Asperger's. It made *all* the difference. I did my research, I adjusted my expectations, and I asked myself, "Can I do this? Is he worth it?" In my heart, I heard a resounding, "Yes."

Bill is my Puddleglum. He will tell me the cold, hard truth as he sees it. If my hair color is too brassy, or my breath isn't as sweet as it could be, or if he thinks that it will be boring to come over and watch a movie, he will tell me straight out. He won't make it nice, or lie to me, or tell me what I want to hear. More than once, his not-so-subtle insights have prodded me to try harder to make my life better. For example, I thought we should live together. Bill admitted that he wouldn't be comfortable living with me until I had a specific amount of money saved up. Normally this would raise a red flag and send a single girl scurrying off. But it wasn't because he wanted to steal from me or use me; he needed to know that I was his financial match and economically stable. Some Aspie's want to know their partner is an intellectual or educational equal; for Bill, what's important is the practical, the material, like numbers and finances. So instead of being offended by this, I looked for a better job and found it, and have been able to save quite a bit this year, for the first time in my life.

Bill's candor and honesty are sometimes shocking. His inability to soothe me when my emotions are rattled makes my world a lonely place to be at times. Like many AS men, he can get inordinately angry (though he's *never* violent), and he often shuts down in the face of stress, social discomfort or emotional displays. Though this is not a good way to be, this too has helped me grow—in patience, in knowledge and in compassion. But it's also a constant exercise in self-observation. After all, how secure am *I* in the face of social discomfort? Is my love for him greater than my need to be accepted in certain social settings? There are times when he will say and do things in public that cause people to wonder raise their eyebrows and judge. We've had waiters treat us rudely, family members ostracize us and strangers laugh at us. This is because Bill thinks it's okay to stir his coffee with his finger, it's all right not to come over on Christmas, and it's acceptable to show me the fillings in his molars while seated in a crowded bar.

But mostly, it's his expression that people notice. When he smiles, it lights up a room, but when he sits there silently, looking grim (which is much of the time), it is often out of place and jarring, and makes people uncomfortable. Of this, he is oblivious.

So why do I stay? What is in this for me? I don't have the comfort of a wedding ring, and I am not given flowers or compliments when I need them most. I have almost no emotional security in this relationship. But, besides the fact that I am in love, I believe we are given the people in our lives for a reason. Every person we meet is, to me, a piece of God. I have never been patient. I have never been particularly compassionate about people with disabilities. I have never had the fortitude to stick with something without almost instant gratification. But when I look back at these last years since I've met Bill, past all the tears, all the heartache, I see how much I've grown as a person. He is the yin to my yang, the voice of reason to temper my passion.

In the *Narnia* book, Puddleglum leads the children into the deepest caves of the earth where they overcome an evil enchantment. Though they thought they were trapped there, doomed to stay forever in the dark, they saw a light, and followed it. It turned out be a window, a tiny hole into the world above, to safety. I have plumbed the dark depths of my soul on this journey, with Bill as my guide. I think we are beginning to see a light. The trick now is to keep our eyes on it.

Rudy Simone is a published writer in the fields of spirituality, holistic wellness, and the paranormal. She is the proud partner of a man with Asperger syndrome and is currently writing a book on the disorder, from that perspective. She is also the author of a young adult fantasy novel, a bedtime book, and a screenplay.

The Reward
Rosemary Banks

"Go-to-skoo."

My son is twisting his lips like he is trying to kiss the ceiling. I turn away from brown arms and eyes that beg me to say the words back.

But I'm not going there with Diop this morning.

I see my autistic son, his gaze a convoluted mix of ebullience and panic.

After giving birth to Diop and his twin sister, Nzinga, I believed that unconditional love would follow like breast milk. But instead our lives became a series of trials through which I learned that until you are confronted with severely life-changing situations, you can never know the extent of your capacity to love.

Here his little happy-ass is again; laying an inch-square picture of a yellow school bus on his shirt on the ironing board. I raise the steaming iron to avoid burning it. We've been through this so many times before.

"Come on, D, the bus will be here in a minute."

He holds up the picture. "Go-to-skoo." I pretend to ignore him. He is garrulous with PECS, the acronym for Picture Exchange

Communication System. PECS is supposed to be especially helpful for children with autism who struggle to articulate almost everything, like my son. But Diop is mostly working my nerves with it.

"Go. To. Skoo," Diop says, again.

"You're gonna get burned, Buddy."

I place the iron on the washing machine so it will not fall off the ironing board, which he will bump as he stomps into the next room, shouting, "Football on Fox, football on Fox." Diop remembers catchy phrases from television or radio, or something somebody said, and uses them as his own private word stock—totally out of context.

I'm rushing. Trying to iron another shirt for him to wear to school this morning because the one I laid out last night is too small. The Risperdal the neurologist prescribed three years ago to help his hyperactivity caused him to gain a couple of pounds each month. Now he's nearly one hundred and fifty pounds. Thank God, at eight years old he's already five feet tall.

The fact that I'm getting him ready to go to school means nothing to Diop; he needs to hear me say it. Which I would've been happy to do if that would end it. But in seconds he'll be back in my face asking me to repeat, "Go to school." It is so irritating I can't take it. So, I give in.

Today is Saturday morning. Nzinga is watching cartoons and Diop is playing Nintendo, turning it on and off to hear the theme music. I'm reading in bed. Nzinga runs in, drops the mail on the bed, and runs back to her cartoon. Among the bills is a formal-looking letter from Diop's school for children with developmental disabilities. *What now?* I think as I tear open the letter.

"Congratulations," it reads, "Diop Banks has been chosen student of the year."

I'm immediately pissed. How fucking patronizing can they be at this school? He takes up a sheet of paper to write his four-letter name, and he's student of the year? Come on. But what really pisses me off is the ceremony next Saturday afternoon. How is Diop going to sit through an awards ceremony?

Lately, it seems I'm always on some level of profound irritability. Deep down I am still angry at God and the world about who my son turned out to be. I breathe, deeply, put on some semblance of a happy face and go tell Diop. "Guess what, Mr. D. You've been chosen student of the year at your school." I hug him.

He pushes me back and says with urgency, "McDonald's, please."

I roll my eyes. "No McDonald's for breakfast. Nice try."

I promised Nzinga we'd go to the movies today because I didn't take them last week for one reason or another. It's probably best that we don't go anywhere today, either; Diop has been having bowel movement accidents the whole week, at school and at home. I was disgusted. He'd worn pampers until he was five, special big hospital green ones from a medical supply company. Even now I wipe him after each BM.

Going to see movies has become a brand-new exciting option for us—one of the public places we can now go like regular people without Diop acting inappropriately. Diop is obsessed with necks. To touch or stare at one intently is a thrill for him. He'll walk up to strangers and try to touch their necks, so I always hold his hand. At the theater, Diop will sit somewhat still and quiet as long as we have popcorn and drinks. After that he starts shouting out embarrassing things like, "Wheel of Fortune, Pat Sajak, gingerbread, cheeseburger, New Mexico."

We're watching a kids' movie, *Juwanna Man*, which Nzinga thought Diop might like because it's a comedy about a basketball team. Everything is going okay. Diop is whispering, "cheeseburger, gingerbread." We're laughing. Then we hear Diop grunt. *Please God, let him just be clearing his throat.* I hold my breath, keep my eyes on the screen, but I'm listening intently for Diop. I hear the grunt again. The reflection of the screen flickers across the pained faces of Nzinga and me. It's as though we're in a movie, and watching one.

"Deee-op," Nzinga scolds.

What to do now? Should I take him to the women's bathroom and try to clean him up with people staring at us? And how could I clean him? Take off his soiled underwear and throw it in the wastebasket and return him to the theater with Diop wearing no underpants?

I look at Nzinga, sitting dejected with her shoulders hunched, her little brown hands folded. To have twins so completely different is a blessing and a curse. I will never give either what they need. "Fuck it, watch the movie." I sit back.

"Mom, don't say that word."

"I said *love it*, watch the movie."

Diop grunts again. I look at my son. His handsome face scrunched, eyes almost shut to little slits. His hands grip the arms of his seat. He pushes, and finally sighs. Desperation washes over me like a hot flash. I think of how much easier my life would be without this fat young boy with curly black hair and dimples. *My life wasn't supposed to be like this.*

For the student of the year ceremony I decide to get Diop a suit and tie, or a dashiki and matching kufi, but as always things do not go according to plan. Divorce and single parenting were followed by poverty. While I'm trying to shop for these things at Deptford Mall, the car breaks down like it does every month. I turn the key to shut off the motor but the key comes out and the motor stays on—there goes the money for something special for Diop.

The Saturday of the awards ceremony has arrived too fast. At least Diop's BM problems have been resolved. His new medication was the problem, and once we abandoned it the daily accidents stopped as well. Now I'm thankful to only wipe him after the standard BM.

The car is good to go, even though smoke from burning oil billows out the tailpipe like some abominable genie, and it loses power if I try to go over forty miles an hour. "Look at the huge puffy white clouds, Mom," Nzinga points at a brilliant sky. I had forgotten the sky, trees, flowers—that it was spring melding into summer. "Yeah, girl," I smile back, thankful she is oblivious to our wretchedness. Diop stops sucking his thumb and jumps into the conversation, "Pat Sajak." Nzinga and I burst out laughing, we know what Diop will say next and we say it with him with exact intonations. "And Van-na White." Diop grins and rocks back and forth. For this moment, away from public gaze, I love my children madly—we are a family.

We find a seat in the midst of faculty and aides from Diop's school. I didn't realize this was a regional event and that Diop's school had selected him as their representative. Diop starts squirming almost immediately. One of the aides gives him a Star Wars book. His teacher Ellen is one of the best he's had since he started school at two and a half. She is a pale, slim, middle-aged woman—intelligent, confident and unassuming. I can see that dignity is the intent as each child is introduced by the emcee. Diop is lying on the floor, kicking the chair to hear the metal vibration and humming loudly. One of the aides takes him for a walk.

With Diop gone I pay closer attention to the program. I'm distinctly aware of the open show of feelings from the children. There are no defenses among them, which is what we all fear as parents—their vulnerability—yet, it's so damn refreshing not to hear blasé, clever comments of cynicism and sarcasm.

A young boy steps forward, throws his arms up and shouts into the microphone in the dialect typical of Down's, "I am the greatest," like Ali. Without thinking, I'm starting to smile. What a great spirit he has. I'm startled to find myself actually feeling the joy and pride these children are showing, as though some small window of vulnerability from my past has been jarred open without my intent. I start to clap harder, proud for each kid.

A young girl with curly black hair and green eyes approaches the microphone with her mother; her father stands behind, intense, wearing a yarmulke. She pauses before talking, as she looks at the audience, the same way we are all looking at her. I can't help thinking to myself that a normal person would not have dared stand in front of an audience and take the time to acknowledge our faces. We with so-called intelligence try to efficiently whiz through most every event in our lives.

The girl smiles into the microphone, and as our audience anticipation peaks she breathes, "Wow." When she adds nothing to it, we clap out of politeness, but also from *wanting* to understand.

Diop is back and almost immediately they call his name. "Our student of the year from Gloucester County Special Services is Diop Molefi Banks. Diop is an African name meaning 'scholar.' He loves school. Everyone hopes that someday Diop will learn how to play the drums—so he'll stop beating on the desk. Ladies and gentlemen, Diop Banks."

We go to the front of the auditorium with Diop walking his boyish, gangling strut (the way comedians do when they imitate retarded people) between his teacher and me with Nzinga on my other side. Diop starts clapping. Clapping is one of my son's favorite pastimes: he wakes in the morning applauding sunrise. Unexpectedly for Diop, the audience claps with him. He is baffled that unlike Nzinga and Mommy, who tell him to shut up already, people have actually joined him.

I say to the audience, "Diop thanks you and Nzinga and I thank you so much," and step back. Holding Diop and Nzinga's hands before them, my spirit feels awakened and uplifted.

Rosemary Banks has a master's degree in creative writing from Rosemont College and in liberal studies from Rutgers University. Her short story, *Being Zarathustra*, has been nominated for publication in *Best New American Voices 2009*.

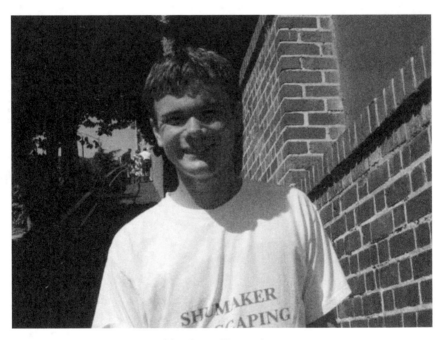

Matthew Shumaker

Love Lessons
Laura Shumaker

It was February 16th; two days after the Valentine's Day storm paralyzed the Northeast. I had just finished my continental breakfast—a rubbery muffin and weak coffee—at a mediocre hotel near the Philadelphia Airport. My flight from Oakland had arrived late the night before, following hours of delays, and I was tired and jittery. I was on my way to pick up my 20-year-old son, Matthew, who is autistic, at his special school in rural Pennsylvania. He had been begging me to take him to Washington D.C. since he'd enrolled at the school three years before, and I thought it would be fun to go over the President's Day weekend break.

When the storm hit I almost backed out, but maternal love and guilt pushed me forward. Sending Matthew to a residential school was the last thing that my husband and I thought we would ever do. But it was absolutely necessary.

Matthew always wanted to be something he can't be: a regular guy like his two younger brothers. In fact, Matthew didn't just want to be a regular guy, but *the* guy—the poisonous plant and weed expert, and the lawn care authority of our northern California community. He would often be seen at our local hardware store with his large hands wrapped around a bottle of weed killer, studying the label intently. My socially awkward son would

approach strangers with warnings about deadly nightshade, ole-
ander and water hemlock. Some would snicker and walk away.

Just a few days into his 16th year, Matthew decided that he should
drive a car like a regular guy, and drove my car through a wall in
our garage. There were other close calls. During his freshman year
at high school, he observed a guy pushing his girlfriend flirta-
tiously and then tapping her on the head. When Matthew tried the
same move with too much force, I was summoned to his school to
find him crying in the principal's office. "Joe did it to Sue, and she
liked it!"

Just when we thought things were calming down following that
incident, a letter arrived from an attorney asking us to contact him
about a bicycle accident involving Matthew. Matthew had col-
lided with a young boy on his bike the month before.

"Matthew," I asked him, "what's this about a bike accident?"

"Who told you?"

"Someone sent me a letter. Was the boy you bumped into hurt?"

"Pretty much"

Dear God.

"Was he bleeding?"

"Probably. Am I in trouble?"

It became clear that Matthew was no longer safe in the community where he had grown up, and his impulsive actions were putting others in peril. He needed more supervision, more than we or
the local school could provide. So we searched for the ideal facility for him, and found this one in Pennsylvania.

My other son's words played in my head as I approached
Matthew's home. "Matthew would be really good looking if he
wasn't autistic." As unkind as it sounded, it was true, and still is.

Matthew is very handsome, with a tall and solid frame, broad shoulders and sandy blonde hair. His eyebrows arch dramatically to frame his brown eyes, and his jaw is square and masculine. But his exaggerated expressions and awkward body carriage make him stand out in a crowd. His forehead twists with intensity, he smiles too suddenly and his hungry-for-friendship gaze is desperate. And he insists on trimming his own bangs, with unfortunate results.

When I arrived at the home, Matthew was waiting on the porch. He smiled widely as I pulled into the snowy driveway of the house he shared with two other students and his house parents, Dawn and Lazlo. That old familiar lump made its way back to my throat. It was clear that he had just cut his bangs again, another botched job. He was wearing jeans, black snow boots and a thin T-shirt, even though it was only 28 degrees. He was blowing the snow with the leaf blower that I'd given him for Christmas.

"He's been so excited about this trip," Dawn said as she loaded Matthew's bag in the car. Matthew had been unusually aggressive about making contact with "hot" girls when his school group went on outings, using suave pickup lines such as "Can I touch your hair?" and "When was the last time you had a seizure?" When counselors from the school tried to offer suggestions of more appropriate exchanges, Matthew yelled, "Stay out of my business!" The pretty girls had scattered, rolling their eyes, and leaving Matthew angry and inconsolable. I applauded anyone who tried to crack Matthew's socially awkward behavior, but I was losing hope that Matthew would ever be able to enjoy the relationship that he craved.

The drive from Pennsylvania to Washington was stressful as I swerved to avoid shards of ice, remnants of the storm, that flew off cars, trucks and tree limbs. Matthew seemed oblivious to my angst and played Beatles music loudly, replaying the first 30 seconds of "Octopus's Garden" over and over each time we entered a new state. By the time we got to D.C. I was ragged and hungry. While I was thrilled to see the Washington Monument, the White House and the Jefferson Memorial for the first time, I worried that it was all too much for Matthew, who was smiling but flapping his hands and rocking double time. We found a pizza place (Matthew's first meal while traveling must be pizza), and Matthew settled down after eating his cheese pizza "with nineteen French fries on the side" before heading back to our hotel for the night.

During breakfast the next morning, I bit my lip as Matthew leered awkwardly at our attractive young waitress while ordering three Belgian waffles and a side order of sausage. "First time in D.C.?" she asked, "You have *got* to go to the Botanical Gardens! Look," she said, pointing at our map, "It's just about six blocks away, right next to the Capitol."

"I'm smart about gardens, I tell you," Matthew said earnestly, trying to impress, "and you should stay away from oleanders. They're poisonous." The waitress rushed away, stifling laughter, leaving me with the heavy feeling in my chest that mothers get when people laugh at their children.

I panicked when I first saw the enormous glass conservatory that housed the botanical gardens and the swarm of people streaming in. Clearly, this was a popular week for middle school tour groups in Washington. A pack of girls in their early teens was bunched in front of us, giggling uncontrollably.

"Those girls are hot!" Matthew said loudly enough to elicit wary looks from the chaperones.

"They're too young to be hot," I shot back nervously as Matthew pushed towards the entrance. "Stay away from them or you'll get in trouble."

"Let me go in first," Matthew said, still eyeing the young teens. "I don't want people to think I came here with my mother."

"That's fine," I said. "But Matthew, this is Washington D.C." I pointed at the pair of armed security guards at the entrance. "It's important that we stay together and use our best manners. Do you understand?"

"If I don't use my manners, will they think I'm a bad guy?" Matthew asked, raising his brows slyly.

"They might. You're a big guy, you know how to behave."

I tried to suppress the sinking feeling that I'd already lost control of the day, that this entire trip had been a bad idea, that the reward for my sacrifice would be heartache for me and frustration for Matthew. It had been easy to fantasize about this trip from California, where the magnificence of Washington was uncluttered by snow, crowds and hot middle school girls. But here we were, at the entrance to the Botanical Gardens. I had to try to make our day a successful one.

Matthew followed the group of young middle-schoolers past the security guards, darting through a series of automatic sliding doors that separated the collections of plants. He was working so hard to distance himself from me that he looked suspicious, and I looked like an undercover agent tracking him. This was not a good place to be running after an oddly behaving son, and I caught Matthew by the arm just as a security guard started marching toward us.

"Is everything all right here?" he demanded. "My mother keeps following me," wailed Matthew. "I need some space. I want to be independent!"

"Of course you do," said the guard, glancing at the hacked bangs that explained all. "But you need to stay together while you're in this building."

Gripped by his desire to connect with pretty girls, Matthew took off again once the guard turned his back, and I followed until he raced through the exit and turned to me, stomping his foot. "Stop stalking me!" he yelled, echoing the words he'd heard directed toward him so many times before. I felt like the young mother whose child was having a meltdown at the grocery store—if only I could just pick Matthew up and disappear into my minivan. Instead, I had to remain calm.

"I have a great idea," I said, "Let's drive to Virginia! You've never been there before."

"Or we could go there first," Matthew said, pointing to the Capitol Building. There was a line curving around the imposing marble steps, also protected by armed security guards. I took a breath. "Can you promise to stay with me and walk slowly," I implored, "and will you remember that this is the most important place *in the world* to follow the rules?"

Fortunately, the line that led to the entrance of the Capitol was moving quickly. It wasn't until we got to the security checkpoint that I learned we were in the line for the gallery that overlooked the Senate floor. There was a special Saturday session debating the Iraq war. Matthew and I were led into the second of three rows that overlooked the Senate floor, where John Warner was speaking. No walls, no bulletproof glass…just open air and the Senate floor right before us. A camera crew was taping the proceedings for CSPAN. Then I noticed five very good looking college-age girls seated in the row behind us.

God help me…

The hot flashes I'd experienced before were nothing compared to the *whoosh* of heat that rushed through me now. Matthew promptly got down to business, leaning back and flirting loudly and awkwardly with the co-ed behind him. She shook her head and motioned for him to turn around, which he did with a sly smirk.

"Talking is not allowed here," I whispered firmly. "I'm serious."

"OK!" he yelled. I glanced at the security guards. Matthew had gotten their attention. What would they do if he erupted again? Just as Carl Levin rose to speak, Matthew twisted around again, tapped the knee of another girl behind him and waved at her.

"Cut it out!" she whispered, then looked at her friends in disbelief. While I was frantically thinking of a way to coax Matthew out peacefully, the girls got up and left in disgust. Matthew rose to leave with them, but one of the security guards motioned for him to stay seated. Matthew looked surprised, hesitated, then sat down and faced forward. His face turned red, and tears poured down his face. Diane Feinstein made her way to the podium. I looked pleadingly at the security guard, and he came to my aid. "Let's go, son," he said kindly, his arm outstretched, and my sobbing son and I filed out of the gallery.

Once outside in the hallway, Matthew confided to the security guard that he wanted a hot girlfriend because he was healthy. I put my arm around Matthew's shoulder and we left the Capitol. I wondered what I could say about this experience that would make sense to him. The obvious explanation would be that since 9/11, it was more important than ever keep a low profile. But how in the world could I communicate that to a person devoid of common sense?

"Those girls really hurt my feelings," Matthew said as we exited into the cold. "They weren't nice."

"I know, Matthew, but you know what? One time when I was your age, something like this happened to me, too."

"Really? Where were you?"

"Well, I was in church, and some really cool guys were sitting behind me. I decided to talk to them."

"Then what happened?"

"I started to talk to them and they told me to shut up!"

"Then what did you do?"

"I started crying. Then my mother, your grandma, walked me out of the church."

"Was she angry with you?"

"No, she knew that I felt bad because the boys yelled at me. She explained to me that at church, you are not supposed to talk. And the boys knew that and didn't want to get in trouble."

"Oh." Matthew was quiet for about a minute, and wiped his runny nose on the sleeve of his pale blue sweater.

"But Mom" he asked, his voice quavering, "did the boys actually think you were nice?"

"I don't know," I said. "I never saw them again. But later there were other boys who thought I was nice."

"That's good. I'm done talking about the girls now. Can we have lunch in Virginia?"

We headed toward Virginia, and as Matthew cued up "Octopus's Garden" on the car's CD player, it occurred to me that this silly ritual had a purpose: it distracted Matthew's heavy, longing heart. As littered with roadblocks as it was, Matthew's search for a meaningful relationship, his need to be a regular guy, was as important as anyone's.

I looked back wistfully as we drove away from the Washington Monument and Jefferson Memorial that we wouldn't visit.

I'll see them next time.

Laura Shumaker is the author of the forthcoming memoir, *A Regular Guy: Growing Up With Autism* (Landscape Press 2008), and a regular contributor to *NPR Perspectives*. A columnist for *The Autism Perspective*, her essays have also appeared regularly in the *San Francisco Chronicle*, the *Contra Costa Times*, the *East Bay Monthly*, and *Hallmark Magazine*.

Navigating the Other World
Todd Caldwell

Guessing at the motivations of a mind that is different from your own rarely works. As a person with Asperger syndrome, I know this very well.

I wonder about the feelings of human connection. I know the instinct to connect with others exists within me; I will feel an emptiness and an urgency. When I do, I will seek out a family pet to play with or hold. Hold it, mostly; the tactile interaction works better for me. I will also seek out conversation, either online or with people at work. It reduces the purpose of connection—to get to know you better—to something I can understand.

When I was a child, the frustration of being unable to connect led to tantrums my family never understood. I screamed and screamed and was sent to my room. I buried my face in my pillow, crying "Nobody loves me" over and over. I would fall asleep crying but wake up fine. I eventually grew accustomed to the frustration and developed a tolerance for it.

My instinct for connection weakened in time and was replaced with an effort to identify the patterns of human connection. I studied how a person acted towards another and its effect on that person, and I tried to recreate the interaction to experience the effect. It never worked. The artificiality was obvious. Even when the other person wanted the connection, it never really occurred.

I still try to force the sensations, though I have given up trying to enlist others to help create them. Attempts at connection from others feel like an intrusion to me, and I know that if they think a connection has formed, I will destroy it through thoughtlessness. So I try to apply my very few successes to any new situations, to borrow the pathways.

I have never felt sadness at a funeral. I have never felt good either. I felt nothing even at the funeral of my favorite grandmother. I saw the expressions on the faces of my aunts and uncle; I watched them hugging each other. I thought to myself, "A blue dress is a good choice. She liked blue. But she needs peppermint candies." She had been in the hospital for a week before she died. I felt something during that week but nothing strong enough to stay with me. During the ceremony, I replayed in my mind the funny eulogy I wrote for her. Writing the eulogy helped. I considered mentioning this at the funeral, but I knew that would be selfish. It would have been turning the event into something about me.

I do have some emotional memories. Two stand out clearly. The first was watching the Academy Awards acceptance speech for the Holocaust documentary *One Survivor Remembers*. I remember the emotional effect, but none of the words, an unusual experience for someone who can recall decades-old dialogue. I have seen the speech twice online since then and still remember nothing of it. But I call on the memory when I see someone in pain and must affect the correct tone.

The second memory is of the death of a beloved pet. She had a benign tumor in her stomach that burst and she bled internally. We rushed her to the vet before she was gone. They prepped her for surgery, but she died before she got to the operating table. The suddenness and immediacy of the event and the adrenaline in my system broke my barrier, and I felt genuine mourning. I hold onto the memory, and use it to help create proper behavior.

This year, my cousin was diagnosed with cancer. My family has been strongly affected by it. I call up the death of my pet and try to lay it like a template onto my perceptions of my cousin. I picture his face. Actually, I picture a picture of his face. Photographs are static, and I can hold images longer in my mind. I try to associate the emotion I felt for my pet with my cousin. I imagine worst case scenarios again: I wonder how he will look and act at the holidays; I imagine the expression on his mother's face; I imagine the effect on his wife and son; I picture him in the hospital; I picture his funeral. I still feel nothing. I wonder if people will notice and yell at me for it. They don't know I have Asperger syndrome. I doubt they would understand even if they did.

I know my parents love me. I know it as absolutely as anyone can know anything, but I cannot reciprocate. I don't feel any kind of pain from this; it is more of a curiosity to me. I know they would like to hear me tell them "I love you," even if I was lying, but I can't. I can't lie, and telling the truth would be rude. But it bothers me.

Of all these situations, the one that bothers me the most is my inability to feel good when someone else does well. It's more than that: I feel angry towards them. I feel betrayed. I know it's wrong, and I know it's due to insecurity, but I can't change it. It's not like being honest when the truth would hurt or saying something wrong when someone needs comforting. With these, I can step back and stay silent and let the normal people handle it. This is a situation where saying nothing causes pain, and there is nothing I can do to prevent it.

There is a positive side to this. I don't feel peer pressure or mass hysteria. I don't accept a lie as the truth. I don't feel much of the pain that fuels the lives of normal people. I react to people based on who they are and what they are like, not on arbitrary details like race or gender or subjective details like religion or politics. It is in cognition and propriety that my interaction exists. Knowing about Asperger syndrome, studying it, has helped. Like a problem to be solved. It's better I try to solve my own problems than to have others try to do it. I guess, because I don't know what I'm missing, I can't really say if or how much it hurts. I have only my imagination for that.

Todd Caldwell lives and works in the Midwest. His writing has appeared in a local newspaper and two short story anthologies. In 2007, he was diagnosed with Asperger syndrome and attention deficit disorder and he works steadily to improve his condition.

A Study in Hope:
A Mother, Her Son, and the Doctor Who Helped

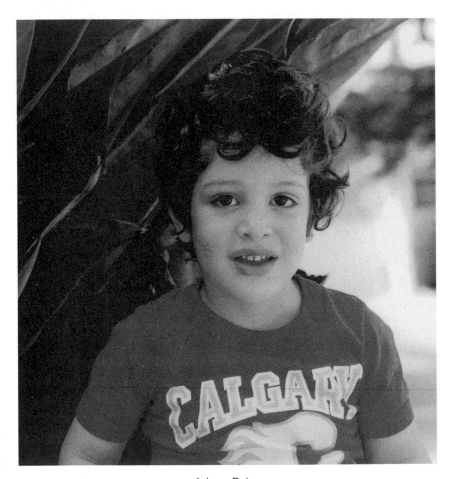

Adam Price

Adam's Journey

Susan Price

I remember clearly the crisp fall day over seventeen years ago when my subconscious whispers of concern became shouts of panic. My beautiful, year-and-a-half-old son, Adam sat on my lap as we rode the Travel Town train in Griffith Park. Excitedly, I made repeated attempts to direct Adam's attention to the vibrantly colored zebras nearby, eager to show him real-life examples of the creatures in his picture books. But regardless of how much I pointed and cajoled, Adam's gaze was elsewhere, spacey and disengaged from both our lively surroundings and my prodding.

It wasn't that I hadn't noticed anything like this before. I had, in fact, seen signs of it, when he didn't respond to his name, made only fleeting eye contact, and flapped his hands at odd noises. I had also been growing increasingly anxious at his lack of language, especially when we were among children of the same age who were gaining words in leaps and bounds. He had what I call "selective deafness," often seemingly tuned out to what was happening around him. It was very confusing, especially since Adam was my first baby and I didn't know what to expect. He was a happy, cuddly, spirited little guy with a head full of soft brown curls and huge, sparkling, chocolate brown eyes to match, always with a delightful smile on his face. His early proclivity with puzzles, letters, and numbers showed us he was bright and his hearing, despite numerous ear infections and courses of antibiotics, was normal.

It was the trip to Griffith Park, however, that finally prompted my husband and me to seek some answers. Our initial consultations with Adam's pediatricians and developmental specialists were inconclusive: his physical and cognitive abilities were on track, we were told, and his language skills, while low, were still within the normal range for a toddler. He could be speech delayed or even aphasic, but it was too soon to tell. We were advised to work with him on identifying objects at home, expose him to lots of kids, and be patient. But we grew restless as his language and social development floundered.

When Adam turned two, we began speech therapy with a very animated and supportive therapist whose approach always began with an object Adam delighted in, such as an apple. She used repetitive vocabulary to describe the apple and how he was eating it, and taught us to temporarily withhold items he wanted while coaxing him to say their names. When Adam finally asked for "muh jhoo" (more juice) at 28 months, we were ecstatic!

However, despite his progress in speaking, glaring problems still remained with his understanding of language, his interest in other children, and his flexibility in routine. He had great difficulty connecting with other children, preferring instead to focus on objects and noises. Garage doors and squeaky gate hinges were big favorites. Walks to the park had to proceed along one particular path only. If we took a different route, he threw a temper tantrum. In addition, Adam's voice had a flat quality, much like a child who was hearing impaired.

Our attempt to integrate him into a private preschool at age 3½ failed because he isolated himself socially from the other children. His speech therapist referred us to an educational psychologist, who recommended that we request an assessment for special education services in our local public school district. They, in turn, devised an "individualized educational program," or "IEP," for Adam and advised that he be placed in a communication-handicapped public pre-school classroom.

This was also the point at which we were told that Adam fit the pro-file of a child with "PDD-NOS" or "pervasive developmental delay, not otherwise specified," a disorder that placed him at the mild end of the autistic spectrum. I remember wiping away the tears as I learned that Adam faced the prospect of a lifetime with a serious chronic condition that would affect every aspect of his social, behavioral, emotional, and cognitive development.

Over the next several years, many other labels would be officially and unofficially tossed in Adam's direction. He was at various times thought to have Asperger syndrome, sensory input dysfunction, attention deficit, high functioning autism, and mixed receptive/expressive language disorder. Our educational psychologist gave us the helpful advice that focusing on what Adam needed, rather than the labels people gave him, was the most constructive way to tackle the problem; the labels were only as good as the doors they opened to help him succeed.

And so began our campaign to help our son transform himself from an impaired little boy to a young man of promise. Speech therapy was the critical "door opener" to this process, providing him with a basic knowledge of language with which to connect to the world around him. Adam's entry into the special education public pre-school program was another very important strategy for beginning his school career in a supportive setting specifically for children with communication problems. Socially, Adam's awareness level was lower than most of his classmates. Among the challenging behaviors he presented to his teacher and aides were pushing other students for attention, slithering on his belly around the classroom floor when he was overwhelmed, and wandering around at recess reciting sto-ries to himself. Academically, he had many strengths: his reading and numerical abilities were well above age level. However, the most complicated, time-consuming, and overwhelming challenge by far was teaching Adam appropriate behavioral and conversational skills that would allow him to effectively relate with other people.

One essential step we took to socialize Adam was a behavior modification program (known nowadays as "applied behavior analysis") that we began through the Center for Autism and Related Disorders (CARD). This therapy, which took place primarily in our home, systematically addressed major areas of social deficit by breaking them down into short exercises or "drills." The drills were administered by various therapists working under Dr. Doreen Granpeesheh, our psychologist at CARD, who designed them to raise Adam's interactive skills and encourage socially appropriate behavior. Over the course of two years, from ages $4\frac{1}{2}$ to $6\frac{1}{2}$, Adam practiced 32 drills which were introduced to him gradually and then set aside as he mastered them. If an old problem resurfaced, an earlier drill was brought out of retirement for reinforcement. When he responded to an exercise correctly, his reward could be anything from enthusiastic praise and smiles to playing a game he loved or eating an apple. If Adam was uncooperative, his punishment would be the absence of those rewards, regardless of tears and tantrums.

Adam's program covered a wide assortment of areas critical to developing his interactive and play skills. It included work on verbal imitation, puppet games, attention and eye contact, proper use of pronouns, asking questions, conversing, recognition of emotions and facial expression, the use of correct tenses, gross and fine motor tasks, creating stories, good sportsmanship and more. Some exercises were designed to include other children and adults, but most were one on one with the therapist. Trips to the neighborhood park, where Adam was prompted to initiate contact with other children, were also part of his program.

Adam's love of board games was an effective tool for teaching him how to cope with changes and interruptions, an especially tough area for him. The therapist would purposely stop a game in the middle or play it a slightly different way, which initially caused Adam to have a "meltdown." Eventually, he realized that the game would be resumed if he accepted the interruption without protest, and he enjoyed the lavish praise he received for permitting a new approach to the rules. Overcoming this difficulty was of immense help in allowing him to get along with peers.

By the time Adam was a first grader, he had made remarkable advances in all aspects of his development. Speech and behavior modification therapy had provided him with a very solid foundation that permitted him to function successfully both at school and at home. Although he was classified as a special education student, he was fully included in the regular classroom and did not require an aide.

Despite the fact that my husband and I were thrilled with Adam's progress, we recognized that there were still differences between him and his peers that posed problems in forming friendships. Adam had a tendency to speak too loudly and to narrate to others rather than converse with them. He had a very literal interpretation of the world which interfered with his understanding of jokes and abstract concepts. Fellow students regarded him as being very smart, but rather odd and spacey. Needless to say, these behaviors impeded his ability to connect with others.

To meet these challenges, a "fine tuning" process began: a master plan to help Adam learn subtle social cues to the point at which he could have a true, reciprocal relationship with another person and blend in with the other kids. It was a lofty goal! Building friendships can be hard for anyone, let alone someone with compromised social awareness. The next ten years were a series of steps that I liken to peeling an onion, removing communication barriers layer by layer and advancing to the center. The frustrating part was that even as we made progress, Adam's peers were maturing as well, which meant that we were always trying to catch up!

The most powerful method in our socialization "tool kit" was keeping Adam exposed to other children as much as possible, besides his interactions at school. Our other son, Sean, who is two years younger than Adam, has been invaluable to him as a friend, role model, and playmate. It was Sean who first taught his brother the joys of companionship with another child and demanded more of Adam's attention as he got older. In addition to Sean, lots of other children, most of whom we met through school and the park, provided further important connections. When Adam invited them to our home, we always made sure to have plenty of toys and activities available. By volunteering at Adam's elementary school regularly, I got to know his classmates quite well and helped him develop relationships with those who approached him with kindness and interest. During play-dates, I tried hard to stay in the background as much as possible, only quietly intervening if Adam started to drift away from the others or was not interacting appropriately.

We also encouraged Adam's involvement with activities that developed his self-confidence and provided interests in common with his buddies. Three of these are particularly noteworthy. Karate taught him focus, balance, physical endurance and body awareness. Boy Scouts gave him positive role models to emulate, a love of the outdoors, goals for community service, leadership training, and, ultimately, the rank of Eagle Scout. Playing the clarinet in his elementary and secondary school orchestras showed him how a group of musicians can create a beautiful sound by working as a team. All of these are activities that Adam continues and which have brought him a great sense of accomplishment and camaraderie.

Despite the times that Adam was teased or shunned by other students, we were determined to give him the chance to grow up in his home community with the same group of kids. We used these negative incidents as opportunities to help him learn how to deal with unkindness, an important survival skill. It wasn't easy to make him understand that the smiles and laughter of others were sometimes at his expense. We rehearsed various retorts to tormentors, although we agreed that, usually, ignoring nasty comments was probably the best response. Fortunately, the majority of Adam's associations with his peers were very positive. Classmates were impressed by his math skills and became accustomed to his longwinded style of speaking. As the years passed, Adam's relationships with his closest pals taught him the value of friendship and compromise, and how to take pleasure in their successes as well as his own. My husband and I formed tight and lasting attachments with the parents of many of our son's playmates. A sort of "village upbringing" developed which provided lots of moral support and "inside information" as to how everyone was getting along. These valuable early friendships provided a strong framework upon which Adam would eventually cultivate other relationships. All of this was made possible by allowing him to attend his neighborhood schools and share a long history of experiences with the same children and their families.

As Adam got older, it became increasingly important for him to monitor his own strengths and weaknesses. To help build his social awareness, we sometimes reenacted awkward situations that came up when he played with his friends and asked him how he could have handled things differently. We were careful to keep our powwow sessions private and to emphasize what he'd done right. We also talked about ways his buddies could have improved their own behaviors and what they may have been thinking.

Sometimes we had to come up with unusual solutions to help Adam control his behaviors. During his kindergarten year, Adam persisted in giggling at odd noises which no one else found humorous, an irritating habit both at school and at home. Asking him to stop only made it worse. I realized that a more empowering approach might work. I told him he could smile at a funny noise, but the second he felt a laugh coming on, he should keep it inside by covering his mouth. This method worked like a charm and it wasn't long before he no longer needed to cover his mouth.

Another technique involved using a video camera when neither he nor his playmates noticed my presence. I was able to catch instances when he was being loud, bossy, or spacey with his friends, as well as times when he was tuned in and appropriate. We watched the tape together after his buddies had gone. I kept my remarks to a minimum, focusing only on the positive moments of the play-date. Adam, however, was his own worst critic! Seeing himself from the perspective of another person, he was surprisingly quick to point out what he should have done differently to make things go more smoothly.

Several times during Adam's elementary school years, we enrolled him in social skills groups recommended by friends or therapists. One of the most effective groups was run by psychologists who created a twelve-week program for children who had trouble making friends. Each lesson had a different theme, such as how to compliment others while playing a game, how to read body language, and how to sustain a telephone conversation. Each child's homework was to call other kids in the group regularly, gradually chatting for longer periods of time. Other groups were led by speech therapists and emphasized how to ask questions, listen carefully to responses, and build a full conversation.

Another important part of Adam's socialization was teaching him to be respectful of other people's feelings and to have a strong sense of fair play. We talked a lot about facial expressions and emotions. We also worked on how to walk alongside another person while speaking to him, a difficult concept for Adam, who thought that the purpose of walking was simply to reach a destination. Consequently, Adam's likeable nature made him easy to be around despite his "differences," and people usually went out of their way to accept him.

As Adam entered adolescence, he had to deal with the sarcasm, innuendo, and wisecracking so prevalent in teenage and adult conversation. He faced the difficulty of having friends who were very bright like he was, but who also had sophisticated senses of humor which he lacked. His brother, Sean, assisted him greatly with this, introducing him to satirical television shows and books. The joking and razzing that took place around the family dinner table also helped. Adam eventually learned that it was okay to smile or laugh even when he didn't quite understand the humor, a tactic we all use on occasion.

During middle school, Adam sometimes felt isolated from his pals as friendship circles and class schedules changed, and new classmates who picked up on his differences made snide remarks. However, by this time, his self-confidence and desire to succeed were strong enough that he could navigate through the rocky early teen years to high school, a much happier experience for him. By then, he had tested out of special education and was doing very well with a challenging course load. I kept open channels of communication with his teachers, usually by e-mail, in case any problems arose. They told me that, although Adam still took longer than most to get to the point during class discussions, his classmates respected and liked him and had long since become used to his circuitous way of speaking.

Adam is now excitedly preparing to attend a wonderful university in California where he will be a statistics major. The friendships he has had since elementary school remain very important to him and he enjoys many large group outings to movies, bowling, and dinner. Although he is not yet dating like some of his buddies, he is very philosophical on that topic. "Everything I've done in my life has always been a couple years behind my friends," he tells me. "I think that going out with girls will follow the same pattern." From what I know of Adam, I think it will.

Susan Price lives in Malibu, California, with her husband, Jonathan, and their two sons. She earned a doctorate in dentistry from the University of Southern California in 1981 and presently works part-time at a pediatric dental practice. She enjoys giving dental presentations to preschoolers and kindergarteners in the area and has written a booklet for apprehensive and special needs youngsters, *My Visit to the Dentist's Office*. Much of *Adam's Journey* is drawn from a guide she created for parents of children with high functioning autism, based on her own successful experience with her son.

Long Time, No See

Adam Price

When I was very small, there were some people who thought I was always going to need special assistance in my life. I think of them as weather forecasters who mistakenly predicted rain when it was really going to be sunny. I far exceeded their expectations and proved them wrong. I am about to start a new life in college, where I will have to develop new friendships and survive on my own. I'm looking forward to that!

I view myself as someone who has looked at the world in two very different ways. I used to have what I call a "holistic" approach to my surroundings. All objects, including people, had the same degree of importance to me. I was just as interested in counting the number of dots on the ceiling as I was in listening to door hinges squeaking or people talking. I also had a special connection with maps, and became quite fond of the direction North because I liked its position at the top of the compass.

The idea of friendship had a very different meaning to me back then. A friend was someone who happened to want to do what interested me. I did not follow my friends when they chose to do something else; I would just go off on my own. Also, if I didn't understand their conversations or their jokes; I would find myself drifting away.

However, I always recall enjoying having other kids around, even if I was on the sidelines.

As the years of therapy, school and play dates went by, I began to see the world in a new, "person centered" way. It was a very gradual process, picking up speed as I went through elementary school. At the beginning of 6th grade, a big change occurred. Since there wasn't any playground equipment on the middle school campus, I had no choice but to spend my lunch periods talking to friends. This was hard to get used to at first, and I would often pass the time kicking the poles lining the outdoor walkways to hear the metallic sound it made. Eventually, though, that habit grew tiresome, while talking to my friends grew more enjoyable. I took a lot more interest in their feelings and opinions. It started to matter to me if I was excluded from a conversation; I wanted to be a part of it.

I became curious about the way my friends perceived things compared to the way I did. I wanted to know what it was like to have the mind of a "typical" person. I often posed puzzles to them such as, "See that tree. I think it's green. You think it's green. But is my view of green really like your view of blue or red or purple?" My friends would tell me that they didn't know. This question led to others and eventually my friends became tired of answering them. Sometimes they responded in annoyance, "I don't know, Adam!" and backed away from me.

It finally occurred to me that the only way I could really understand and blend in with my friends was to work harder at observing and copying their behaviors. I spent time contemplating why my friends held longer conversations with one another than with me. I sometimes became frustrated with my mother for letting me know that I appeared "tuned out" in social situations, because I already noticed this myself.

I also realized that my confusion with humor and sarcasm interfered with how I related to my friends. I worked hard to overcome this. The toughest part was learning what made a joke or phrase amusing. For example, at first I couldn't understand why saying, "long time, no see" after having just seen someone, was considered funny. I practiced this phrase and others, but my timing was always off. I was constantly waiting patiently for the perfect time to say something funny, but I would end up interrupting people and no one would laugh.

It wasn't until a scouting trip to Hawaii during my 8th grade year that I made a breakthrough with my friends. During a pause in conversation, I made a joke that fit right in with our discussion. Everyone responded with laughter and one friend even remarked that he had never heard me tell a joke before. I was so excited! This experience made it clear to me that timing was everything.

That same year, I was finally released from my resource program. Up to that point, I had been in special education. Yet, it wasn't until I was nine years old that I began to wonder why I had to be separated from the rest of my class for speech and resource help. I found it annoying that I often had to leave during math, my favorite subject. Sometimes, my speech teacher had to persuade me to go with her. My resource class was a separate period so that I wasn't pulled out of other classes, and I was embarrassed to tell my non-resource friends where I went during that hour. I felt that people weren't seeing my full potential because it looked like I was less capable than I really was. I felt underestimated, even by my own parents. I knew I was socially delayed, but I believed I could fend for myself and get help if I needed it. At the end of middle school, I made absolutely sure that I gave 110% effort to my comprehensive three-year evaluation for special education. I wanted my examiner to see who I really was and what I could accomplish. I was beyond triumphant when I learned that I no longer qualified for services.

It still takes me longer to process what I read and to organize my thoughts on paper. For this reason, my parents requested a Section 504 classification for me during high school. This is a federal law that gave me certain accommodations if I needed them. For example, I could ask for extended time on exams, books on tape, or front row seating in class. At first, I felt uncomfortable asking for any accommodations; I was being "different" again. But my chemistry instructor talked to me about the importance of being a better advocate for myself. I followed her advice and spoke up when I needed help.

I made the decision to enroll in Advanced Placement United States History as a junior, even though my parents were worried it would be too much for me. This course required a lot of reading and three structured essays a week. I took this challenge to improve my reading comprehension and writing skills (I also happen to like history). The course was even more work than I imagined, but I learned a lot about argumentative writing. Most importantly, I learned I could take on my weakest area and still succeed.

I pushed myself to take several other AP classes, too, the most important of which was Calculus BC. This course was taught by a fantastic former college professor who had written many calculus textbooks. He made me feel so good about math that I decided I would like to major in math or statistics in college.

When I look back at my life so far, I have two opposing feelings. On the one hand, I would like to repeat it as a typical earthling who never had to face being different from the rest of the population. I recall many painful moments when I would ask my mother why I was born with difficulties that my friends didn't have to face. On the other hand, I believe that my differences allow me to think outside the box and come up with new ways of approaching problems. I've also learned how to keep on going when things get tough, which is why my mother claims that the Eveready Bunny and I have a lot in common. Besides which, my years of special education and therapy evaluations prepared me well for enduring those tiring SAT and AP exams.

I try as much as I can to look at the positive side of this whole experience. It has indeed been a long journey for me to get to this point: a graduating senior. Yet, it is not over. While I have been successful in making friends, keeping them, and learning how to communicate better, I now have to put my skills to the test in college. I am eager to start fresh in a place where no one knows my beginnings and I will be treated like everyone else. Only after I have made it on my own, will my journey be complete.

_____

Since writing this essay, Adam Price did, in fact, put his skills to the test and is now happily attending a California state university where he is an honors student majoring in statistics. He is also a clarinetist in the university wind orchestra, participates in three social clubs, and has made many new friends while he still prizes his old ones.

Applied Behavior Analysis and Autism

Doreen Granpeesheh, Ph.D.

and Jonathan Tarbox, Ph.D.

Autism is a disorder characterized by deficits in social development, which is the ability to understand social information and to use that information to interact with others in a meaningful way. Because each child with autism is so different, the difficulties they experience with social development are also very different. On one hand, children who are more severely affected by autism may completely lack the ability to play or interact with others. Such children sometimes have no interest at all in others and may prefer to spend their time alone, engaging in repetitive activities. On the other hand, children who are less severely affected, like Adam Price, may have a genuine interest in having relationships and may spend a large amount of their time trying to interact with others. These children are sometimes referred to as having "high-functioning" autism or Asperger syndrome, or they may be children who were once severely delayed but "caught up" through intensive behavioral intervention. What we often see in these children is a genuine desire to cultivate friendships and social relations but major difficulty with doing so.

Oftentimes this difficulty can be traced back to the child's inability to understand the perspectives or mental states of other people. This understanding is often referred to as *perspective-taking* or "Theory of Mind." Perspective-taking is critical to successful social behavior, and a lack of perspective-taking ability is the primary stumbling block for many high-functioning individuals with autism. Many simply do not understand that other people have mental states different from their own, and if one cannot understand someone else's perspective, one cannot possibly hope to make and maintain a meaningful social relationship. The primary areas of perspective-taking that are critical to interacting effectively with others are as follows:

First, to effectively interact with others, one needs to be sensitive to their emotions. One must be able to identify when another person feels happy, sad, angry, scared, etc. For example, the way in which you might greet a friend who is crying is quite different from how you might greet that same person when they are smiling. Getting these two completely different situations confused will very likely make your friend feel unsupported or misunderstood. Put simply, successful relationships depend on *behaving differently* in the face of different emotions.

Second, one must be able to understand and respond to the relatively long-term preferences of others. For example, if your friend hates dogs and has always hated dogs and you buy her a book of dog photographs for her birthday, this will not help maintain your friendship.

Third, understanding and responding to momentary shifts in preference, sometimes called "desires," is crucial. For example, when having a conversation with a friend, it is important to be able to identify when your friend is bored with the topic so you can consider changing it. Children with autism will often continue talking about the same topic over and over, without realizing that the friend they are talking to is getting bored and therefore doesn't want to talk to them anymore.

Fourth, social relationships require the ability to understand the *sensory perspectives* of others. For example, talking to someone on the phone about something that is directly in front of you but that the other person cannot see will not be effective unless you understand they can't see it and you tell them what it is. Very young children often make this mistake; they will say to the person on the other end of the phone something like, "Look what I have! Isn't it great?" Children with autism often will not develop the ability to figure this out, even when they get older.

Fifth, understanding others' knowledge is foundational. For example, if your friend already knows that you just bought a new video game system, telling him that fact again will not be a good conversation starter. Instead, you might talk about a new game you played with the machine or what game you want to buy next. This subtle but important difference is based upon your understanding of what your friend already *knows*. The ability to tie sensory perspectives and knowledge together is also very important. In the course of our everyday social interactions, we need to be able to infer what other people know, based on what we know they have seen, heard, tasted, etc. For example, telling your friend that you bought a new puppy yesterday is not necessary if your friend was with you when you bought it. In short, understanding the general concept that seeing something leads to knowing about it is key to successful social interaction.

Sixth, social functioning requires understanding the difference between *knowledge* and *beliefs*. If you *know* something, you have a fair degree of certainty that it might be right. However, you may *believe* something that could be false. Understanding the difference is important to successful social interaction. For example, if your friend tells you that he has a favorite treat at his house and, upon arrival, it turns out that it was already eaten, it's important to be able to understand that your friend believed it was there but that he was simply wrong to believe it was still there; that is, he was not trying to trick you or lie to you. It is also important to understand that different people have different beliefs and that it is okay for others' beliefs to be different.

Seventh, successful interaction requires understanding others' *intentions*. On a daily basis, people do many things that affect one emotionally but that effect depends on the actor's intention. If you do not understand the intention, then you cannot possibly respond appropriately. For example, children in the hallways of schools bump into each other frequently, simply due to the number of children crowded into a small hallway. A child with autism may not understand the concept of accidents and interpret it as another child intentionally trying to hurt him. Being able to figure out other peoples' intentions and then respond appropriately is a critical skill that won't necessarily develop in children with autism.

Finally, understanding *deception* is critical for social interaction. Many "typically" developing children develop a problem with lying that must be addressed directly, but many children with autism suffer from the opposite problem—a complete inability to speak anything but the truth. Of course, we don't want our children lying constantly, but the ability to withhold certain aspects of the truth is crucial to successful social behavior. For example, if you don't like your friend's new haircut, it won't do very well for your friendship to bluntly point that out to them when they haven't even asked you. Most children's games and most jokes depend on deception at some level as well. When you "give away" the punch line when telling a joke, the joke is not funny anymore. The humor in the joke depends on withholding information about the punch line until just the right time.

Children with autism often lack these basic social cognition or perspective-taking skills. Experts disagree on the cause of this deficit and scientific research has not yet provided a clear answer. However, it is clear that this it is often not a problem of intelligence. It is very common for a child with autism to have an average or even advanced level of intelligence but still not have the ability to understand others' perspectives. It is also important to understand that it is not just a matter of motivation. Many children with autism honestly want to be able to interact with others effectively and are genuinely sad when their attempts at making and maintaining friendships fail. After ruling out both intelligence and motivation in many cases, we have realized over the last 15 years or so that it is simply another skill that needs to be taught.

We are fortunate to have at our disposal a scientific approach to successful skill teaching that has evolved over the course of 40 years of careful scientific research and clinical development: Applied Behavior Analysis (ABA). ABA is the applied branch of the science called Behavior Analysis. Behavior Analysis is a science of learning and motivation. More than 100 years of research with humans and animals has demonstrated that a small number of laws of learning and motivation apply to the behavior of virtually all organisms, including humans. ABA uses these basic laws of learning and motivation to fix socially important problems; autism is one of the many areas addressed by ABA and it is currently the best-known approach to treating the disorder.

The ABA approach to autism involves analyzing exactly which skills a child needs to learn and exactly which challenging behaviors need to be replaced. *Positive reinforcement* procedures are used to teach new skills. Everything that a child with autism needs to learn is treated as a skill that can be taught, including daily living skills, language, social skills, academic skills, motor skills, perspective-taking, and advanced cognition. Each skill area is broken down into very small, teachable units and is taught gradually. Each child's unique strengths are built upon in the gradual process of attempting to teach everything the child needs to know in order to catch up to his or her typically developing peers. Some of the better-known procedures used within ABA are Discrete Trial Training, Incidental Teaching, Pivotal Response Teaching, Verbal Behavior, and Positive Behavioral Supports. All of these approaches are based on the same principles of learning and motivation, and all require advanced training in the science of ABA. Modern comprehensive ABA programs for children with autism include some elements of each of these procedures.

ABA does not teach only rote behavior; rather, it is a comprehensive science, based on fundamental principles of learning and motivation. Behavioral research has focused on the two basic areas of learning: rote learning and generalization, with the intention of discovering exactly how people learn by rote and exactly how they form generalized concepts. This research has allowed present-day practitioners to teach rote behavior when needed (e.g., every single time you want to cross the street, look both ways before you do it) and how to teach generalized concepts when appropriate (e.g., understanding other peoples' beliefs).

In essence, the ABA approach to concept formation is to teach many, many different examples of the concept to be conveyed in many different settings, with many different people, all the while varying everything in the teaching situation except for the particular details of the concept. For example, if you want to teach a child the concept of "yellow", then you teach her to name many, many different yellow objects, each object being completely different, except for the fact that it's yellow. Exactly the same procedure is used to teach perspective-taking. You teach the child to talk about and understand someone else's mental state, given a particular situation, and you teach the same mental state over and over, all the while varying everything about the situation (e.g., person, time of day, cause for the mental state, etc.) except for the particular mental state. Through this process, a person learns to ignore the irrelevant details and forms the actual concept by attending to and understanding the details that actually form the basis of the concept. In other words, the person learns to generate "rules" that are flexible and can be modified according to the different details they experience in any given encounter. These rules can then be applied to future, similar encounters and can provide assistance to the person in identifying how to behave in a socially appropriate and acceptable manner.

We first met Adam when he was 4½ years old and attending pre-school. He was a very proficient reader and excellent at math concepts as well. However, he was unable to hold a conversation and had a great deal of difficulty socializing with his peers. Although his classmates were amazed at how bright he was, they were confused by his inability to make meaningful connections with them. He was genuinely interested in his peers and wanted desperately to interact with them but could never find the words or figure out how to enter their worlds and become one of them. Although Adam had made tremendous gains in basic speech and academic skills, he had difficulty understanding other peoples' mental states and with being able to adjust his own way of interacting based on them.

One of the first mental states we started working on with Adam was that of understanding other peoples' emotions and the various details related to them. We started with showing Adam pictures depicting people displaying various emotions, in situations that likely caused the emotions, and then encouraged Adam to talk about the situation. For example, we showed Adam a picture of a child who just fell off his bike and was crying. In a natural conversation about the picture, we asked Adam questions like, "How does he feel?" to which we taught Adam to respond "Sad"; "Why does he feel sad?" to which we taught Adam to respond, "Because he fell off his bike," etc. When Adam wasn't sure, we would give him hints. When Adam gave the correct answer, we would give him positive reinforcement by praising him or doing something fun with him, like playing a board game.

We also helped Adam generate some rules. For instance, we taught him that people usually smile when they are happy and frown or even cry when they are sad, and that some situations may make one person happy while making another person sad. We repeated these same processes but with different materials until Adam was able to answer correctly across a wide variety of emotions and with new and different materials that he had never seen before, thereby demonstrating that he actually understood the concept and that he hadn't simply memorized particular behaviors. We then moved on to more advanced concepts, such as asking, "What could you do to make the child feel better?," "What would make you feel better if that happened to you?," "What would make Mom feel better if she was sad?," and so on. To further ensure that the skill we taught had resulted in genuine concept formation, we tested it by setting up situations in real life where other people (friends, family, etc.) displayed emotions and we watched to see whether Adam was able to respond effectively in the natural setting. Additional examples continued to be taught until he no longer needed any help and could genuinely apply the concept across every aspect of his daily life.

Understanding the emotions of others is important but it's not enough on its own. So we proceeded to teach every other aspect of perspective-taking with which Adam demonstrated difficulty. A very important one was *sensory perspective-taking*. We started by testing Adam with "false belief" tasks. For example, when one of our therapists was alone in a room with Adam, they would open a box, place an item in the box, close it and then invite Adam's mother into the room. Then we asked Adam, "What does Mom think is in the box?," to which he responded by telling us what *he* knew was in the box. In other words, he did not understand that what he saw allowed *him* to know what was in the box but that, since his mother was not there to see it, she could not possibly know what was in the box. We used the same basic strategy for teaching sensory perspective-taking that we used with emotions. We started small, made it easy for Adam to be very successful right away, used lots of positive reinforcement, and gradually increased the difficulty of the tasks, all the while teaching across many different examples and situations to prevent rote learning.

Soon enough, Adam was able to distinguish between his own sensory perspective and that of others and he was able to use that understanding to then infer what other people knew and believed. We then used the same basic strategy to teach Adam everything we could think of that was related to preferences, desires, intentions, thinking, knowing, deception, and eventually to tie it all together. The basic approach was to try to identify everything that might be related to the ability to understand someone else's mental states, assume it's a teachable skill, break it down into small parts, and teach it, bit by bit, until there was nothing left to teach.

Of course, a great deal of Adam's success had to do with the support he received from his family. Every time we worked on a particular area, Adam's mom made sure Adam had ample opportunity to practice the skill involved with other people, in novel situations and under varying conditions. She also helped him form these concepts or rules by prompting him, guiding him, and encouraging him to think about his experiences.

Each child is different, of course, but in cases like Adam's we are very frequently able to completely remediate a child's lack of social cognition, thereby giving the child the ability to understand and interact more effectively with others. Our work with Adam and the work we did with many others like him at that time was exploratory, because no one back then had specified how to actually teach these skills. Since then, we have put much time and effort into analyzing every detail of how to teach social cognition to children with autism and have created clear and easy-to-use teaching programs which have been integrated into our everyday approach to teaching children with autism.

It is very encouraging to find that the same basic process, of breaking complex cognition into small, teachable skills, works in teaching other areas of advanced cognition skills, such as *executive functioning*, which is essentially the skill set required to pay attention to the relevant aspects of a situation, to plan, problem solve, monitor one's progress toward a goal, and tie it all together by adjusting one's own behavior based on how one is doing in achieving the goal. It turns out that this area of cognition can be taught as a skill, too.

Last summer, we were delighted to have Adam join our team at the Center for Autism and Related Disorders. He spent three months as an intern in our Information Technology Department and was admired and liked by his colleagues. Adam has continued to grow and has become a very thoughtful, friendly, and considerate individual. He attends college now and is an "A" student. He is very intelligent and hard working and will undoubtedly enjoy a healthy and successful future. Adam's case serves as a great example of the tremendous gains that can be made when ABA is started early and done well. Adam is also a shining example of how complex cognitive skills can be taught, just like any other skill, by using a careful, systematic, ABA approach. It was an honor to be able to work with a child as unique and fascinating as Adam and it is a great pleasure to watch him mature into the man he has become today.

We are proud of Adam and the hundreds of children like him who have flourished in our practice. These children are our shining stars and their success brings hope to thousands of families with newly diagnosed children today.

Dr. Doreen Granpeesheh is the Founder and Executive Director of the Center for Autism and Related Disorders (CARD) and President of the Board of Autism Care and Treatment Today (ACT Today). She is a psychologist and board-certified Behavior Analyst and has been providing behavioral therapy since 1979. She received her Ph.D. in psychology from the University of California at Los Angeles and is licensed by the Psychology Board of California and the Texas State Board of Psychologists.

In 1990, Dr. Granpeesheh founded The Center for Autism and Related Disorders (CARD) and through its 17 offices located around the world has provided diagnosis and assessment services and behavioral treatment for thousands of children with autism and related disorders. In 2005, she founded Autism Care and Treatment Today, a nonprofit organization that provides support and funding to families of children with autism. In addition, Dr. Granpeesheh is a principal member of the Thoughtful House Center for Children, a charity organization that provides behavioral services in collaboration with medical treatment and research. Dr. Granpeesheh is a member of the Defeat Autism Now Executive Council, and is on the Scientific

Advisory Board of the U.S. Autism and Asperger's Association and on the National Board of the Autism Society of America. She is recognized as one of the world's most prominent experts in the treatment of autism.

Dr. Jonathan Tarbox is currently the Director of Research and Development at the Center for Autism and Related Disorders. He has worked in a variety of positions in the field of behavior analysis, including basic research, applied research, and practical work; with individuals with autism and other developmental disabilities of all ages and their families and care providers. He has worked for and in public school districts, private schools, sheltered workshops, group homes, developmental centers, behavioral consultation agencies, hospitals, and community-based recreational programs in direct service provision, supervision, consultation, and program development and director roles. His early career included positions at both the New England Center for Children and the Kennedy Krieger Institute. Dr. Tarbox received his Ph.D. in behavior analysis from the University of Nevada in Reno, under the mentorship of Dr. Linda J. Parrot Hayes. Throughout his career in autism and behavior analysis, Dr. Tarbox has been actively engaged In research in applied behavior analysis and has published several research articles in peer-reviewed journals, as well as book chapters in behavioral psychology texts. Dr. Tarbox's current research interests include recovery from autism and teaching complex language and cognition to children with autism.

Part III
Finding Shelter

A Sestina for Michael Johnson
Michael Johnson

My name is Michael.
I am autistic
Try as I might there is no speech
My thoughts come out slowly with typing
Yet they come quickly in my head
Don't judge me too fast
Others move and talk quite fast
But give no thought to Michael
They use their mouth not their head
With no understanding of what it means to be autistic
Slow down and wait for the typing
These words on the screen are my speech
Why is there no speech?
The thoughts come fast
They bottleneck with typing
and don't show all that Michael
has to say. Because I am autistic?
Or because my hands move slower than my head?
How can I express all the things in my head?
When there is no speech?
How do I conquer being autistic
when the world moves so fast

that there is no time for Michael
to fit in his typing?
I spend hours a day typing
Yet I get only a part of the thoughts in my head
Many things you don't know about Michael
The thoughts are lost with no speech
Let's slow down, I can't type fast
Please don't forget the autistic
Many things are hard for the autistic
Friendship is not easy through typing
The society of friends moves fast
Which direction will they head?
So much is done with speech
Others will talk, not so with Michael
Michael is more than autistic
No speech, wait for the typing
My head is moving too fast

An Aspie's Guide
to Everyone Else
Jason Seneca

AS is considered by most people, experts included, to be a very mysterious disorder. Not surprisingly, people with Asperger's tend to view normal society as mysterious and dangerous. Articles on "tips for living with an AS family member" and "coping with the Asperger's patient" abound on the Internet; however, I have seen very little in the way of advice to the AS person attempting to cope with the rest of the world.

To help fill this void, I have prepared the following list of assumptions and misunderstandings that, in my experience, people with Asperger's and high-functioning autism commonly make concerning "neurotypical" people (NTs).

As a person who has Asperger syndrome, I am not attempting to justify antisocial behavior or to portray my fellow AS'ers as victims of an intolerant society (I actually believe that most people with AS enjoy certain advantages over the average person). I only hope that my experiences with and observations of both AS people and NT's can help to explain some of the confusion that people with AS feel when dealing with normal society. To those of you who do not have AS, perhaps the following will give some insight into how the other half (~0.4%, actually) live. To those who do deal with the condition on a daily basis, this is written for you.

1. Most NT's consider their emotions to be a source of relevant data.

NT's consider emotional experience as relevant, or more relevant, than objective observation. I'm sure you've heard phrases such as, "It feels like the right decision," or "I feel good about this choice." This tendency is not a product of ignorance or weak will. Emotion is simply more valuable to NT's than to people with Asperger's. When considering a decision, they value and consider the emotional outcome as well as the practical one. As such, they require both emotional and practical data in order to make an informed decision.

2. Words are not enough.

I've often found myself thinking, "How can this person not know how I feel? I've said it a million times!" Remember that emotional communication is a part of almost all human interaction. The presence or absence of emotional cues is widely considered to be a fairly accurate indicator of a person's sincerity. NT's place large amounts of trust in their abilities to perceive and interpret emotional cues. Because of this, they have a tendency to place their trust in other people according to their interpretations of emotional cues. If you find yourself having to voice how you feel over and over again, you are probably not giving off the appropriate impression. It's not that your friends or loved ones don't trust you when you talk about your emotions; it's that you look untrustworthy to them. It is important to find alternative methods of expression.

3. Emotion is always justified.

Emotions occur spontaneously. They are the products of millions of years of evolution. Their triggers are buried deep within our neurology and history. As such, we cannot blame or draw judgment on anyone for the emotions that they may feel. The true measure of a person is in the way he or she reacts to and deals with emotions. Considering this, it is not appropriate to think,

"He has no right to feel that way," regardless of how illogical the feeling may appear. We know that NT's have less control over their emotional experience. We should allow them the space that they need to feel as they must.

4. For most people, emotion is not a purely personal experience.

Emotion is the glue that binds individuals together and identifies members of the society to one another. These bonds are constantly reinforced by the exchange of emotion. Emotional commerce reassures people that they are not alone, that they are surrounded by trustworthy people of like mind and intent. It seems rational to describe emotion as a form of social currency, the medium of exchange in human interaction. A person experiencing emotion changes his dynamic within society. His value in the social economy, the give and take of emotion that occurs in nearly all human interaction, is drastically altered. The value of his social currency changes.

In my experience, AS'ers simply do not change in the same way. When I am angry, I know it. I feel my heart race and my vision narrow. My muscles tighten. My voice takes on a harsher tone. The fact that I feel anger is undeniable. I have learned, however, that my anger does not manifest itself in a way that is easily understood by NT's. I simply don't "look" angry or "act" angry, and only those closest to me can discern when I am truly upset.

Like most AS'ers, I experience anger on two levels. The first, physiological and primal, is described above. The second level is cognitive. I understand that I am angry, that my anger is affecting my thoughts and ability to interact with others, and that I must exercise reason in order to avoid mistakes. From this perspective, anger seems distant, more of an abstract concept than a tangible event. Neither of these levels of experience has obvious outward signs. This, it seems to me, is the very crux of Asperger's: the inability to synthesize emotion and cognition. The average person seems to make this connection innately. Indeed, I suspect that a very large majority of people have never considered that the presence of an emotion and the experience of that same emotion can be separate.

In interacting with an AS person, the emotional, NT person feels cheated. In return for emotion, he may receive advice, humor, money, or physical assistance, but he does not receive the form of payment that he expects and desires: reciprocal emotion. It is as if he sold a car and was paid in jellybeans. The jellybeans may be worth as much as the car, but he has no simple method of redeeming their value; they are worth less to him. His annoyance with the AS individual is not irrational. Within the framework of the social economy, it is justified.

5. Helpful advice is not always helpful.

If you're like me, you cannot count the number of times that you've been rebuffed for giving unwanted advice or correcting an honest mistake. In the viewpoint of most AS'ers, mistakes exist to be corrected; problems exist to be solved. The rest of the population simply does not seem to feel the same way. Understand that, to an NT, virtually all interaction has an emotional element. By making unwanted corrections, we are not only saying that the information is incorrect. We are also saying that the *informer* is incorrect. The connotation is implicit. Often, we see problems to be solved where NT's see experiences to be felt. Thus, when faced with another person's problems (experiences), it is important to clarify whether they seek a solution, sympathy, or merely verbal support for what they already believe. Mark Twain described the trend succinctly: "Advice is what people ask for when they know the answer but wish they didn't." Remembering this when people relate their problems to you can save you a lot of grief.

6. Many NT's prefer happiness to truth.

Don't believe this one? Try a simple experiment. Ask your non-AS friends and family the following question: "Assume, hypothetically, that I had conclusive proof that there is no life after death.

Would you want me to tell you about it?" You may be surprised at the number of people who answer "No." This does not result from a devaluation of truth, or a wish to delude oneself. It is a product of the higher value placed on emotion. In the example above, they would be giving up an enormous amount of emotional well-being to gain a truth that does not directly benefit them. From this perspective, it's simply not a fair trade.

7. Vive la différence!

Accept the fact that there are things about NT's that you may never understand, and things about you that they will probably never know. I am constantly bewildered at the amount of pride that so many people feel toward local sports teams. By contrast, I know very few people who understand my desire to create highly-detailed fictional worlds. I have personally been accused of being cold, shallow, selfish, insensitive, egotistical, repressed, emotionally dead, incapable of emotion, and incapable of love. If you have Asperger's, you have probably been the subject of similar condemnations at times. If you're like me, these accusations tend come as a shock. You know that you are a sensitive and caring person; you see these tendencies within yourself and can identify their outward manifestations. How could you be perceived so harshly?

Are people with Asperger's doomed to walk through the world with pockets full of unspendable social currency? Of course not. We are not emotionally bankrupt. We cry and laugh and rage. We *feel*. Our differences only assert themselves in the subtle language of emotional expression. Should we learn to interpret and generate these nuances? Is it our fate to live lives of constant personal analysis, constant mimicry? I say no. By doing so, we deny ourselves and our true feelings; we limit our contribution to society. We should spend our time and energy employing our talents, not masking our shortcomings. It is my contention that people with Asperger's can hold an uncommon position in society: that of the objective observer. The way in which we perceive emotion and our general position as outsiders of standard social convention allow us a unique perspective of humanity.

AS'ers are poorly equipped to alleviate fear, but well supplied with the tools to identify and eliminate the causes of fear. We cannot rationalize hatred away, but we can rationally find and eliminate the sources of hatred. Without fully experiencing normal emotion, we are better able to manipulate and analyze emotion. I feel that this must be the AS'ers' ultimate social role, the most fitting way in which we can repay our social debts: mitigating fear with knowledge, superstition with rationale, condemnation with hope. We are hardly capable of adding to the strength of our social bonds, but well suited to advancing the richness, diversity, and wealth of our societies. It is to this end that we must direct our talents.

All humans experience and appreciate beauty, kindness, and love. It is on these premises that I relate to the bulk of humanity. "*Love thy neighbor...*" is more than a rule for moral behavior. It is an effective method of relating to the 99.6% of people who do not think as I do. Love works. Don't forget it.

Jason Seneca is a paramedic and writer with Asperger syndrome.

Autism the Beautiful Mind

Elyse Draper

I look into the dazzling amber pools that hold no emotion. I see a boy as handsome as any Christmas gift. At first glance, the figurine is missing something important. The full lips, that will never understand the passion of a first kiss, are painted on by a skilled hand. The ringing voice of a child, monotone, never expressing the love we know is there. You look seven years old, but you've been endowed with the weary, one-word responses of a seasoned war veteran.

You and I discuss the existence of Santa Claus without the mirth or mysticism of your classmates. You turn to your mother, not noticing the yearning for love in her eyes. Her hugs are returned not with an embrace but with squirming to be free. I wish I could give you the joy of being tickled and take away the annoyance at being touched. Your sister loves the boy who reacts to horseplay by lashing out instead of laughing; you have unintentionally given her the gift of patience.

I watch bewitching eyes that see the world in all its grandiose textures, delicate senses absorbing too much stimulation. There is the naive mind breaking under the weight of excessive information; I can see it straining to keep its rigid hold on reality. Your exquisite focus on obtaining order only painfully reminds you that you have no control. When peeking from around the walls you have built, you become acutely aware of the differences between yourself and others.

Can't you see how wonderful you are? No, that would mean you'd have to understand what is happening to you. Why, you don't even understand your own expressions. There is the true sadness of the ailment; your simple angelic beauty and inner light are hidden behind the face of an indifferent child. You stand in front of the mirror making faces to match the pictures in your "emotions" book, and although you can mimic them you'll never truly understand their meaning. I have watched you studying your classmates, trying to understand if you have said something funny or sad, relying on your powers of observation to guide your response. I see the panic as you lose track of the expressions and body language, not knowing how to respond. You can only walk away. Will you ever understand that you put more energy into acquaintances than most people put into marriages? You are magnificent in the attempts at friendship, but that doesn't matter as you walk alone across the playground, head hung low.

I hold this little figurine up to the light... I was mistaken, you're not missing anything... you have extra inside. Oh, what a precious burden to be given this gut-wrenching gift. As I hold you up and look through, as if you're as delicate as blown glass, I can see the prisms of indescribable light projected in fractured rainbows. Innocence, purity, consideration, and confusion intermingling with a genius' gifted mind. You have the most beautiful mind; if we could just learn to be as strong as you, learn to try as hard as you do.

Elyse Draper resides in Denver, Colorado, and has worked with children for over seventeen years, the last two of which with children with special needs, while completing a degree in pediatric psychology. She is currently working on her first book.

God's Special Child

Sheila Webster-Heard

Shifting uncomfortably, I sat in my son's individualized education plan meeting, cradling my one-year-old daughter and trying hard to conquer fatigue. I was near tears and trying desperately to project an appearance of strength. The very first question of the meeting was, "What are Darius's strengths?"

In complete silence sat the principal, the psychologist, the speech therapist and her assistant, along with Darius's teacher, the case worker and the occupational therapist. My seven-year-old autistic son had been in their presence six hours a day for a little over a month, and none of them was able to think of anything good to say about him. Their obvious displeasure showed on their faces and I could feel my confidence waning.

What was I thinking, coming to this meeting without an advocate? I wondered. I had heard the horror stories of parents who were pounced upon, ignored and belittled at I.E.P. meetings, but until this point I had never been a casualty. I thought it was obvious that I was committed to helping my son adjust. I thought they understood when I explained that my child was regressing and his severe behavior was agonizing to me as well. However, to the team of individuals who sat around the table, frowning, my efforts were unimpressive.

"Well...he has a nice smile," the speech therapist offered. I chuckled at her nice gesture, but no one else did. I knew from that point forward I would spend the rest of my time wondering if we had done the right thing by moving out of our public school district to place him in a "better" school district. I knew I would be tormented daily as I relinquished my child to the bus aide and school bus driver, who would then deliver him to the same group with whom I was sitting in the meeting now.

I began to question if this was the right placement for my child, even though it was a school specifically for autistic children. Ironically, I had fought hard to get Darius into the school, where I could be certain the teachers were trained and equipped to handle the challenging behaviors that many autistic children exhibit. Now, I was clearly confused.

Darius isn't a monster. He is a child who has been afflicted with a developmental disability. It isn't his fault that he has a problem with change and that he throws a severe tantrum if he has to wait too long. Darius didn't decide that he would scream in order to communicate his wants and needs. Autism causes Darius's communication deficiencies, and its symptoms were causing the problem, not Darius.

Unfortunately, these expressions of anger and intolerance were all too familiar. I've only been impressed by a very few educators, who didn't let autism obscure their view of the child trapped inside. I cherish the memories of those who used their energy not to debate about medications but to bring about a change in Darius. We keep faith that one day we'll cross paths with other teachers who possess that same energy and passion.

As each attendee commented on Darius's shortcomings and behavioral issues, I couldn't help but think of the child I knew. On the inside, I smiled and thought: too bad none of them has ever seen Darius during the days of summer when we take him to the park. On those days, he's grinning and giggling; his long legs are taking even longer strides, his arms are outstretched as if he's trying to capture the rays of the sun. And too bad none of them will experience those moments when I've stepped into Darius's classroom, watching him work quietly and confidently, and he suddenly looks up at me and smiles, so happy that he can show us all that he has potential. My soul aches for those who are scared off by Darius's autism and will never know that he is creative, intelligent and affectionate.

Pain will always resurface when other people's looks pierce me to the core. But what will always give me solace is knowing there are plenty of wonderful things about Darius. The most important: he is one of God's special children.

Sheila Webster-Heard is a freelance writer and the mother of two sons who are on the autism spectrum. She lives in Calumet City, Illinois, with her husband and three children.

Chasing Chris

Linda O'Connell

During the thirty-one years that I have been an early childhood educator, I have had my share of special needs students. But despite
their problems, not once did I ever regard any of my students as a
"problem child." I learned early on that the way in which teachers
and parents view children often governs the way in which we treat
them. I know many teachers who dread the next school year
because they've been forewarned about troublesome Tommy or
sassy Susie. I say, "Bring them on," to the parents who warn me
about their terrible toddler. I don't buy into the stereotypes. Terrible
twos and threes, frisky fours and fives, no way; these rambunctious
Rambos are just trying to establish their territorial rights: if it's
yours, I want it. If it's mine, you can't have it. If it's in your hand,
I'll snatch it. In a mistaken attempt to control, they make a real
name for themselves: brat or problem child. Those are the typically
developing children. Toss in a few quirks, hyperactivity, language
and social interaction deficits, and a diagnosis of being "on the
spectrum," and you can get a feel for what my days are like.

The autism spectrum is a huge imaginary arc along which children
who have the disorder exhibit symptoms from mild to severe. My
first introduction to autism happened many years ago. Chris
screeched and wailed on his mother's lap as I spoke to parents at

orientation. His mother apologized and said she didn't know why he behaved as he did. It was apparent that this blonde, blue-eyed, stocky little boy was different from any child I'd ever taught. I tried to speak to him, but he avoided eye contact. Many shy children bow their heads and shrink into themselves, but this little boy writhed in his mom's lap and looked vacantly at the ceiling as he screamed.

"He's smart; he really is," his mother said. "He can recite lines from a movie he saw weeks ago. And he can read." I smiled reassuringly and told her he'd be fine. I wasn't so sure about myself. I had no idea what autism was at that time, but I went to the library and researched behavior disorders. All indications pointed to autistic tendencies: deficits in social interaction/reciprocity, language difficulty and distractibility.

The first week of school I discovered a new term, echolalia. If I said, "Chris, come sit here," he repeated verbatim what I said to him. I decided then and there to treat Chris no differently than I would any other student. I expected of him what I expected from any other child his age. I expected him to sit on the floor at circle time each day before being allowed to go to free-play. When he writhed and flung himself backwards, I didn't scold. I compensated by standing behind him, supporting his weight; he could only lean as far as my bony legs would allow. I presented my lesson each day with Chris leaning his head and back against me like a ton of bricks. Upon greeting him every day, I knelt to his level, tapped my nose and insisted on eye contact. When he echoed me, I modeled the language I wanted him to use. I praised his efforts and rejoiced when he was successful without my prompting. During circle time, he would blurt entire episodes from his favorite movies and some days I completely lost control as the students said, "Hey, I saw that video." Some days I threw my hands in the air.

I observed Chris at free-play. He interacted with objects but not people. When he was able to select his own activity, he always chose a parent-teacher *Sesame Street* magazine on my desk. The day he sat down and began to read aloud fluently, I realized that he had already mastered the pre-academic concepts I was trying to introduce.

It was difficult for him to sit for any length of time. It would have been so easy to allow him to wander about the classroom during circle time. But I knew that he and the other students had more valuable lessons to learn than ABC's and 123's. I insisted Chris sit with the group each morning. But fifteen minutes was overwhelming for him. His disruption created chaos.

I came to the conclusion that chaos could actually be a learning tool for the entire group. I explained to the class that Chris couldn't help being noisy and he needed to move, that his body wasn't able to sit as long as theirs. I asked if they had made an effort to play with Chris or talk to him. Everyone tried to tell me at once how they had tried, unsuccessfully. I decided that Chris was entitled to fun social interaction just as every other student was. At some point every day—either when my legs gave out, or Chris became too vocal—I'd close my book, put away the flannel board, shove the shapes into a box and shout, "Okay, Chris, run!" Running was his favorite motor activity. The children watched him zoom around the room flapping his arms.

One day I shouted, "Okay, it's Chase Chris Time!" He screeched with delight; it was the only time his face registered happiness. He laughed and ran like the wind as the students giggled and ran around the very large classroom in every direction trying to catch him.

The special education teacher came to observe him one day. She looked at me in disbelief when she saw him taking off his shoes. Her unspoken message was, *aren't you going to do something?* I smiled at her and said, "He learns best with his shoes off. He takes in information that way." When he began to fidget, she tried to control him. "Chris, sit still and listen." I smiled. "He is listening. But he's unable to sit for very long." I helped him get his shoes back on and then I nearly floored the specialist when I shouted, "It's Chase Chris Time!"

The class went into action. Chris babbled and laughed as the group carefully darted to and fro. Not only did the pre-kindergarteners develop spatial awareness as they avoided colliding, they also learned how to make one little boy with a different learning style very happy. Every single student was able to interact with Chris, and before long he wasn't viewed as being different. He was viewed as being the fun kid in class. The special education team was prepared to assign him to a self-contained classroom, but after observing peer interaction and my consistent approach with him, they decided on inclusive education; they mainstreamed him into my class.

Many days I went home exhausted, but at the end of the school year I decided it had been worth every ounce of energy I expended documenting his language development and social interaction skills. Even the shin bruises from connecting with Chris's back and head were worth it. In May, the specialists noted that Chris had achieved most of his goals and benchmarks, but most of all his language development had improved from 90% echolalia to 50% spontaneous typical language. My greatest reward!

I taught many lessons that year, but none was as great as the one a little boy taught each of us: that we are all special and unique, we all bring our gifts to one another and the world. It is how they are perceived and received that matters. Chris is grown now, but I can still feel him leaning on me. He certainly left an impression.

Linda O'Connell has been an early childhood educator in St. Louis, Missouri, for three decades. She is a published writer; most recently her stories have appeared in *Voices of Breast Cancer*, published by LaChance Publishing, and several *Chicken Soup for the Soul* books. Her essays, articles, and poetry can be found in *Reminisce, Reader's Digest, The Mochila Review, Andwerve, Flashquake, Joyful Woman, Whispers from Heaven*, and more. Linda also writes a bimonthly column for a regional newspaper and teaches a memoir writing class for senior citizens.

The Feast
Colette Porcelli, MS Ed.

The best advice I was given during graduate school was that no two snowflakes are alike, and neither are two children. The lesson to be learned was to treat children as individuals, so you can discover their true potential to learn and grow.

Upon graduation, I felt competent to enter my own classroom as a teacher of special needs children: I had been taught the most up-to-date educational theories and methods and my bookcase was filled with highlighted textbooks covering a multitude of topics on children with special needs. I was advised by many of my professors and peers that, as time passed, I my teaching style would change with the varying needs and energy of the children I taught and the requirements of the board of education. I was also told that I would always need to stretch my ability and be flexible in response to these changing needs.

Over the years, this turned out to be true. Each year my classroom was filled with children with varying needs, learning styles and social skills. Some had been diagnosed with LD (learning disabled) related to their reading, math, and/or writing abilities. Others had been diagnosed with ADD or ADHD Some were labeled ODD (oppositional defiant disorder). And there were a number of children who were autistic and described as PDD–NOS (pervasive development disorder–not otherwise specified).

In the beginning, regardless of the labels that had been affixed to their academic files, these children were, unfortunately, expected to meet the demands of the same curriculum and pass the same series of state exams as all of the other students. Worse, they were expected to co-exist and "blend in" with the rest of the students, who simply did not understand them. To make matters worse, some of my colleagues and supervisors lacked the knowledge, understanding, skills, and compassion needed for working with and encouraging these children with special needs.

As the weeks and months passed, I became frustrated: the mandated material and textbooks rarely offered me room to teach in a way that interested my students—or me, for that matter. I felt there was a part of me missing in my classroom: I wanted the children to feel the energy I possessed, and I wanted to discover their individual academic potential, their learning styles and, most importantly, their unique personalities.

In November of my second year, an opportunity arose to do just that. A parent offered me a turkey she had won in a raffle and I gladly accepted it so that my students, our classroom assistants, and I could enjoy a Thanksgiving lunch together. During our meal, we talked about how next year we could have additional foods and invite others to join in our celebration of thanks.

And that is just what we did. The following year, I started our plans a month in advance and sent out signup sheets for side dishes, decorations, linens—the works. The students began working on invitations, choosing music that would accompany the luncheon, constructing placemats, and they gladly participated in supplemental lessons about the holiday. Through these simple tasks I began to see additional methods I could use in my classroom for holding the children's attention, whetting their interest, and encouraging them to work in groups.

Our turnout doubled the following year and my students were thrilled. We did a write-up about it for our school paper. Most importantly, we generated a list of items that would make the next year's celebration even bigger and better. My class contained at least two grade levels, which meant that many of my students would be present the next year and, better yet, we invited the other special education classroom to join in our newly titled "Feast." Within two years, we doubled in size and in responsibility, but most importantly the children were having fun and learning at their own individual levels.

Eventually, our school year began with preparations of our Feast. Math lessons incorporated calendar countdowns, seating charts, and recipes. Social Studies became part of our daily lessons. I was really having fun teaching and the children were even more excited to learn. I was filling our days with academics while rarely picking up a textbook. Reading exercises exceeded the usual time allotment because the children began to bring in books from home and clamored for a chance to read aloud to prepare for speeches they would make on the day of our luncheon. We were excited to go to the library to learn more about the holiday, entertaining, and cooking.

Each year, the Feast took on a different energy, as did the process leading up to it. Some years the turkeys were gotten in truly interesting ways; in other years the trimmings represented diverse cultures and tastes. I began to involve the occupational, physical, and speech therapists to lead our group lessons related to the Feast so that they too could be part of our celebration and not be confined to seeing my students individually or in small groups. The Feast gave them an opportunity to work with the children in their natural classroom setting, among their peers, and to see them flourish in an activity that was truly, uniquely theirs.

One of the best outcomes was the involvement of the parents. My students glowed with pride when they announced that their parents were coming to organize the Thanksgiving mural or to work on our welcome speeches. Together, we had all found a way around the labels and differences, creating a community of unique learners who were able to work toward the same goal: our feast of thanks.

Fortunately, the theories, labels, and approaches related to educating children with special needs continue to evolve, encouraging us to work harder to inspire these young minds. And as a woman with a love of children and snowflakes, I am fascinated to watch them all change and grow in their own uniqueness as we continue to learn more so that we can better help them.

Colette M. Porcelli holds a master's degree in special education from Bank Street College of Education and has taught in public schools in New York, California, and New Jersey. She is currently at work on a master's in social work at New York's Stony Brook University. Colette presently lives in Westhampton Beach, New York, with her fiancée and their two black labs. They spend their summers playing on the beach, and their winters admiring the snow.

This story is dedicated to her first teacher—her mother Lydia—who encouraged her to learn more about her uniqueness and to see the beauty of the snow.

Sensory Detective

Deanna M. Walsh-Bender, MSEd.

I have never lived more than a few miles from the shore of the Long Island Sound. At times in my youth, when I felt adrift in life, I would make my way down to the water's edge. Its comforting ebb and flow would bring perspective and anchorage as it warmed my soul with a spiritual serenity that I so desperately needed to ease my adolescent hardships. As a teenager, I could never have known that one day my life's work would be to give that same sense of anchorage to others.

In my first year of teaching, I was assigned a student named Samantha. This beautiful young woman was my first encounter with an adolescent with Autism Spectrum Disorder. One of the last patients to have been rescued from the deplorable conditions in the infamous Willowbrook School, she was extremely sensitive to sound and would scream a very high-pitched scream if her environment became the least bit noisy. She was extremely thin and refused to eat during our morning breakfast social. Samantha was also "tactile defensive," pulling away from the slightest physical touch. Even before my training in ASD began, I felt an extreme desire to make her world safe and to make her feel she could trust others. I wanted to discover how to provide her with the same comfort and anchorage that those days at the beach provided to me in my youth.

For hours, I would try to engage her in class activities, such as simply sitting with the remainder of the class or participating in the morning breakfast social or the newspaper assembly line and delivery. Instead, she would stand off to the side, rhythmically rubbing and tapping her fingers, looking out the window and occasionally twirling her body. In an attempt to reach her, I decided I would take time out each day to stand with her, side by side, rubbing and tapping my fingers as well, while talking softly to her about what the class was doing. When she would twirl, I would twirl with her. I did not receive anything I could identify as a response. It seemed no matter how hard I tried, there I was, without the keys to unlock her from what appeared to be a world of isolation and inner torment.

Unknown to me at the time, Samantha, like others with ASD, was constantly challenged by our world. She was continually bombarded with messages sent to her by a brain that received information and processed it inaccurately. Stress and anxiety increased the inaccurate processing of this information, resulting in heightened sensory jumbling and a complete withdrawal into her locked-away world. In reality, she was trying to make sense of a world that was confusing, unpredictable, painful, and very often frightening. Samantha's reactions to the world around her was similar to what is experienced by many others with ASD; reactions often under-recognized and gravely misunderstood.

It brought me great, visceral sorrow to learn that Samantha experienced common sensations as confusing, painful, and frightening and that, along with these challenges, she was unable to comprehensibly communicate with others, which worked to increase her anxiety and stress. I came to find that I was not alone in my empathic response to this young woman: sensory integration dysfunction confused and frustrated many professionals, leaving them feeling unable to assist those with ASD.

Then one early afternoon, an angel walked through my classroom door and blessed me with a set of keys to unlock some of the doors to Samantha's world. This sensitive and loving soul was an occupational therapist who held a special interest in those with ASD. She taught me to be a "sensory detective" of sorts. Once I understood the unique hardships that this sensory integration dysfunction created in Samantha's life, I finally began to feel as if perhaps I could make a difference, and maybe even be that anchor I so wanted to be for her.

I eagerly embarked on my mission to learn about ASD, devouring everything I possibly could on the subject. I began my detective work and set forth on my mission to find the keys to unlock Samantha's world:

Lock # 1: Samantha would not join the remainder of the class because they were too noisy and this was literally painful to her. Key #1: I provided her with a set of soft walkman headphones to muffle and reduce some of the sound. Entrance #1: Samantha sat with the class just about every day for the remainder of the school year.

Lock # 2: Samantha had difficulty with our breakfast social. The students were given various breakfast choices on visual picture boards. They would communicate their choices, set their place at the group table, prepare their breakfast, and learn socially appropriate mealtime behaviors. Key #2: In speaking with Samantha's foster mom, I learned that one of the few foods Samantha enjoyed was peanut butter on crackers. I also learned that she would drink apple juice, but could not tolerate the smell of orange juice, almost to the point of illness. Entrance # 2: I altered the visual picture boards by removing orange juice as a beverage choice and adding apple juice. I also included peanut butter and crackers as an option. From then on, every day Samantha joined in the breakfast social and made independent choices on her communication board. Finally, her voice was beginning to emerge. No longer lost, sitting by the window locked in her own world, she became an active part of the class.

Lock # 3: Samantha couldn't participate in our newspaper assembly line. This was an activity in which the students sat together at the table and collated the daily newspaper as a work-study project. The newspapers were then delivered throughout the building. Key # 3: After extensive "sensory detective work," I came to realize that Samantha could not endure getting her hands dirty and refused to hold the newspapers because the newsprint would soil her hands. I decided to provide her with a pair of soft cotton gloves to wear throughout the activity. Entrance #3: Samantha became part of the working newspaper crew, participating daily without great difficulty.

While Samantha's symptoms regularly ebbed and flowed, she maintained the unchanging core ASD difficulties in cognitive functioning, communication skills, social interaction, behavior patterns and sensory processing. Yet, I found that I made the most progress with her once I learned the role that the central nervous system plays in sensory integration dysfunction. Samantha's inefficient sensory integration clearly contributed to her problems with class participation, learning, and behavior.

One day, in the midst of my teaching the remainder of the class with Samantha's full participation, she silently walked toward me. As she approached, she made direct eye contact, smiled and held out her hands to tap my fingers. From that point forward, whenever I spoke to Samantha she would gaze into my eyes, speechless, but full of expression. Occasionally, she would reach out to take my hand. As I gazed back at her, speaking softly, I desperately wished that she could tell me her thoughts and her dreams. I prayed that the kindness and sensitivity we tried to show her that school year allowed her a sense of peace, just as the Long Island shoreline had done for me.

From that year on, ASD became my passion. This first-year teaching experience formed the foundation for the remainder of my life's work. At age 22, how could I have known that a sweet girl named Samantha would lead me, guiding us both through her lonely world of isolation, floating as we were in a sea of confusion, to a sheltered coast? Thank you, Samantha, for trusting me to point out the anchor, even when the storms railed against us.

I now can no longer observe life without wondering, "What might this sensory experience be like for an individual challenged by ASD? How might they interpret this situation?" Since then, I have had the wonderful opportunity to work with hundreds of students and clients, representative of all points along the ASD continuum; each one uniquely touching my heart. I have also encountered many more dedicated professional angels along the way. I have grown alongside my students and clients, and through their complex way of viewing the world, I often feel they've taught me more about life than I could have possibly taught them. Their dynamic, creative, and spirited voices need to echo loudly throughout society. These voices will emerge to reach the hearts and minds of others as they have so poignantly reached mine. Perhaps, side-by-side, we may anchor each other.

Deanna M. Walsh-Bender has served the autism community for 18 years as a special education teacher and as an autism consultant. She holds a Bachelor of Arts degree in Elementary and Special Education and a Master of Special Education degree in Autism. She will complete her LMSW in Social Work this year. In her private practice, CAPES: Child Advocacy & Parent Empowerment Services, she works with children, adolescents and their families providing consultation, therapy, advocacy and parent education. She lives with her husband on Long Island, New York.

Mario's Shirt

Sherry Antonetti

Having a master's degree in special education meant I had guaranteed job security, no matter what the town. Moving to a new school meant I would be dealt the toughest cases, those that none of the veteran teachers wanted. Now, looking at the IEP write-ups for the six students in my class, I drew a deep breath. The write-ups spoke of behavior problems and self-abuse. The descriptions painted a monstrous picture of the six sixteen-year-olds who would be my responsibility for the next school year.

The educational goals spelled out in the reports had me wondering if these kids were as low functioning as the paperwork indicated. Could watching TV actually be a goal? Did I really have to let a child have private time in the bathroom in order to ensure his good behavior the rest of the time? And how was I going to keep one child from throwing himself against the wall every time I wasn't looking? My teaching assistant was a fifteen-year veteran and she assured me that this class was full of "nasty habits." She especially warned me about Mario.

When Mario was brought to my table on that first day of school, he promptly started gnawing his knuckles and wrists until they bled. I blocked his hand from his mouth. Mario promptly socked himself in the jaw with his other fist. I imagined that the other teachers and my aide, who were watching me, were thinking, "Rookie." Presented with his breakfast, Mario immediately calmed down enough to eat. When breakfast was over, I instructed him to take his tray back to the counter. Verbal prompt, stating expectations, straight from the textbooks, what we're supposed to do. Mario stood. He put his hands on the tray. He laughed. Then he threw the tray across the cafeteria. Nice, I thought.

"You need to pick that up, Mario." He laughed again. I pointed and put his hands on the tray: verbal and physical prompt, again going by the textbook. Mario started slapping his hands on his legs, tuning me out.

"There's nothing wrong with your hands or your legs, Mario. Pick up your tray."

He laughed—at me, I thought. Putting his hands on the tray, I walked behind him, clasping his hands to the tray as he tried to throw it at least four more times. He also threw head butts and got my nose once. He laughed again, and now I knew it was deliberate. He head-butted me once more before we finally put the darned thing down. He bit his wrists all the way to the classroom.

In the classroom, I had a radio on low, playing classical music. Mario pulled up a chair and placed his ear next to the speaker. He was calm. I made a mental note to bring a walkman the next day, and we proceeded with the rest of the morning routine. It was only when I began morning meeting that I noticed his shirt. It was much too tight for him. He lived in an institution and probably didn't get to choose what shirt he wore. I happened to have a few shirts in the classroom for teaching laundry. One of them was a button-down oxford my husband had donated. I asked Mario if he liked it. He touched the sleeve and laughed. I put it on him. He laughed again. But this time it was a laugh of joy that I hadn't heard from him before. We got on with the rest of the school day and the aide remarked that he wasn't gnawing his hands as much. But, when we took off the shirt before bus time, he cried and immediately went back to bloodying his hands. "Guess he was mad at his wrists," my aide joked. But it was true. When he didn't see his wrists, he didn't hurt himself.

Gradually, Mario came to know that the shirt would be waiting for him every day at school, and his wrists and knuckles began to heal. By allowing him to wear a walkman, we also succeeded in getting him to stop repeatedly slugging himself when walking from the cafeteria to the classroom. Carrying a tray was still an adventure for us, though. It was like a battle of the titans! I lost a necklace (and my patience a couple of times) and suffered two nosebleeds from his head butts.

Then, one day, my aide and I were astonished and gratified to see Mario pick up his tray and quietly carry it the fifty feet to the cafeteria counter. Everyone in the cafeteria seemed to hold their breath as he made his way to the dish window. Two inches from the counter, he stopped, dropped his tray and laughed. Everyone in the cafeteria laughed too, even me. Then the real miracle happened. He picked up the napkins, the silverware, the milk carton and the plate from the ground, placed them back on his tray and put the whole thing on the counter. Then he wiped up the mess and laughed all the way back to the table. We clapped, we laughed, we gave him his walkman and Mario looked at us like, "What's the big deal?"

He progressed from there, so well that he got a job delivering papers to the rooms at a hotel. But after a week he was returned to the classroom for aggressive, self-destructive and unsanitary behavior. Had they used the shirt we provided? They had not. Nor had they allowed him to use the walkman when he walked the hotel's corridors to make his deliveries.

Mario was given a second chance, armed with the shirt and the walkman. He did great. He moved on to other job sites with the vocational coach, now aware of the tricks for keeping his self-abusive behaviors in check. The next year, he progressed to a new vocational class, going to a job site every day. We threw a party for him. My aide and I chipped in to give him four button-down shirts and a walkman.

I've long since moved to a new town. If I knew where to find Mario today, I'd buy him an iPod and a new button-down shirt.

Sherry Antonetti is a former special education teacher who now writes humor and spiritual columns and stays home to raise her eight children.

Silent Messengers

Anne Spollen

I met him right after my fifteenth birthday, nearly thirty years ago: the silent, green-eyed boy who moved in next door. Not the kind of teenager who babysat or thought very much about children, I smiled at Daniel as he stood near the hedge separating our houses. After a few times of saying hello to Daniel, I stopped. Daniel did not answer me. He did not look at me. Daniel looked at the hedge; he stood there patting its flat leaves while his mother worked a few yards from him, restoring the overgrown garden in their yard.

"He doesn't speak," his mother whispered to me one day. She had asked me to help her hold a trellis up while she mounded dirt around its base. Daniel sat on the stoop near us, dropping rocks into a pail of water. "No one knows why he doesn't talk yet. I mean, he makes sounds, and repeats words, but he doesn't actually speak in sentences of any kind. Sometimes I think it's because his father isn't around anymore. But I've had him tested more times than I can count. They just don't know, the doctors." I nodded. Daniel kept slipping rocks into the water.

"I thought if I could get a decent garden put in here, he might play more. You know, outside, the way boys usually play. He doesn't play like other kids, either."

I watched Daniel. He hummed softly while lining up the rocks into two perfect paths. Each rock had to be dipped twice into the water. He did not seem to be aware of either his mother or me.

"Maybe if I fix things up around here, he'll play more like a regular kid."

I kept watching Daniel. I had to: I did not want to face his mother after she said that. It seemed to me that Daniel was much further from being a regular kid than a garden and a few toys could fix.

During the next month, Daniel and I silently orbited each another. As the weather brightened, I spent increasing amounts of time working in the yard. Daniel stood at the hedge, patting the leaves. A few times, I tried to catch him looking at me as I planted flowers or painted the rocks edging the path. But Daniel was never looking at me; he looked only at the leaves on the hedge.

One day I took out the red wagon I had played with years back.

"Would you like to go for a ride in this?" I asked.

Daniel kept patting the leaves.

"Hey, did you hear me?"

Daniel stopped patting the leaves. He stood by the hedge, silent as a footprint, staring at the leaves. He would not look at me.

"Let's see then." I thought of my friends who had younger siblings, friends who could conjure games and ideas readily. What would they do? I could not think of a single way to entice Daniel. Then my hand fell on a packet of graham crackers I had put in my pocket that morning for a quick breakfast and forgotten to eat.

"Do you like these?" Daniel's face crumpled a bit as I opened the cellophane. "Definitely, you hear well, so you just don't want to talk to me." I smiled. Daniel looked at me, but not directly: he seemed to look past me, to a place only he could see. I turned. All I saw was the parked car and a cat in our driveway. "What is it?" I asked.

Daniel took the graham cracker. He smiled. This simple gesture, the smile of a four-year-old boy, captured me.

"I'll be here tomorrow," I promised, "and I have lots more crackers like this. Lots."

Daniel did not show the next day. Or the next. I knew his mother worked, and Daniel spent time at his grandmother's on the other side of town. But I hadn't learned yet that the only predictable behavior of this boy was that I could never predict it. Daniel showed on the fourth day, dressed in blue, as always, and began patting the smooth, vaguely clove-scented leaves on the hedge. I held out the crackers. He took some and chewed without looking at me.

"I brought some things I thought you might like," I said with careful casualness. "I found this book about cars."

In truth, I had bought the glossy book at the mall the night before, hoping to see this strangely silent boy smile.

"Cars," he repeated.

"Yes, cars." Only he did not look at the book. He looked past me, once again toward the empty driveway, touching the smoothness of the pages. When he was done, he turned and ran back to his house, leaving the book spread open on the lawn.

"Some kids have speech delays," my aunt, a teacher, told me one August afternoon. "They catch up."

"But there are other things... he doesn't hook into me in any way. I bring him toys, and the only one he likes is a pail. He fills it with rocks, wets them, then lines the rocks up. Sometimes he repeats one word I say over and over, but he never says the word first."

"He'll probably go to a special school then," my aunt said. "But I have never known you to take any kind of interest in a child. What happened to the girl who never wanted children because they would interfere with her work as an aspiring anthropologist? Don't tell me you're growing maternal in your old age."

"No, not yet," I laughed. But I had to admit, Daniel was the first child to have touched me in my life, and I did not know yet that his touch would change the course of my life.

That summer, I spent more and more time with Daniel. He and his mother came into their front yard in the evenings, and while she planted and dug in the abandoned garden, I watched Daniel. And through him, I began to understand him.

Daniel did not like red things. He did not like anything that "crunchled"—a word we made up together to describe the sound that made him put his hands over his ears (cellophane wrappers, paper bags, dried leaves—all examples of items that crunchle). He did like graham crackers, pictures of cars, and walks to the oak tree and back. Never farther, never a different way—down to the oak tree at the corner, and back to his yard. We walked the same path each time, and the routine seemed to comfort him. He would hold out his hand, touching my pinky twice to let me know he wanted to take our walk. I read to Daniel; I tried to teach him the names of colors, but he would not look at the book when I asked him to look. Daniel looked at the book when he wanted to look.

I worked part time that summer, typing in a hot, dusty office for a car rental agency. Each day, as my stultifying afternoons came to an end, I walked home quickly, hoping to see Daniel. Something about getting him to smile made me forget that I did not like my job, that geometry loomed in September, and that my best friend had stopped calling in July. When I was with Daniel, all that mattered was getting him to smile, or better, to hear the strange, growly laugh he gave when anything delighted him. I like to think we filled each other's empty spaces that long summer. But Daniel had done much more for me, I just couldn't see it yet.

That fall, Daniel and his mother moved to his grandmother's house across town. His mother promised to bring him back to visit. I would look out the windows sometimes when I heard the sound of an approaching car, but Daniel and his mother never came back.

I suffered geometry, made a new best friend, and eventually landed in college. That first semester, I sat in a cold dormitory room, highlighting definitions in an introductory psychology book. When I came across autism, I sat up: this was a description of some of Daniel's behaviors. Two hundred miles and three years later, I could still see the clear green of his eyes, still hear his low growly laugh. Autism. I repeated the word out loud. And at that moment I knew; Daniel had shown me. I was not going to be a globetrotting anthropologist as I had written in my college essay. All my plans of travel and discovery would occur on a much smaller scale. Despite my bookish reputation, my apparent lack of interest in children, my aspirations of travel and research, I wanted to learn more about children like Daniel. I wanted to be a classroom teacher. That had been Daniel's silent message. I had not understood it right away, as I had not understood Daniel right away. He had shown me that not everything is—or should be— rushed and obvious. That summer when I believed I had been teaching Daniel the names of colors and the types of cars, he had been teaching me that the kind of truth you learn through time and silence is the kind that matters the most.

After nine years of teaching, Anne Spollen left the classroom to raise her own children and write part time. She is currently working on a second young adult novel about a teenager with Asperger syndrome. Her poetry and fiction have been nominated for *Pushcarts* and her first novel will be released by Flux Publishing in 2008.

I Love Lucy
Brian Lafferty

If someone were to ask me what it feels like to be autistic, it would be hard for me to describe. I hardly ever think about it. In fact, a sportswriter whom my family knows said that he would never have guessed that I am autistic. It used to feel frustrating to be autistic but that has changed over the years. Now I feel really good and consider myself very lucky.

I was eleven years old when I was diagnosed with high-functioning autism. It was confusing for me because I had never even heard of the term before. My parents and teachers knew that I had a learning difference, but in the years before my diagnosis it was believed that autistic people never spoke and isolated themselves from the world. When high-functioning and low-functioning autism were discovered, I had my diagnosis. It was as if my life had been a jumbled jigsaw puzzle, and now the pieces were coming together.

In elementary and middle schools I had a difficult time. Seventh grade was one of the worst school years. I had to deal with a teacher whom my parents thought was the worst any of us kids ever had. She treated me as if I was a misbehaving child, which wasn't true: there wasn't a great understanding of autism among teachers and schools back then and many of my actions were often misinterpreted. Once, I was quoting a line from *I Love Lucy* and a classmate thought I was calling her a name. The teacher wouldn't listen to my explanation and gave me detention.

Like many autistic people, I am very sensitive to loud noise, and once I went into the bathroom to get away from the school band, which was practicing in the next room. The teacher accused me of being defiant and uncooperative. My parents tried to explain it to her and to the staff, but to no avail. The teacher wouldn't even make an effort to understand.

I wound up having to leave that school and enrolled at another middle school to finish off the year. I lost all of my friends, and for the next few years I resented everyone at the school where that teacher had been so unfair to me. It was better at the new school. but the feelings of resentment didn't go away. It was as if the whole world had come crashing down on me. Those feelings have largely gone away. When they do surface, I remind myself of the success that came later.

Things went better at a private school I attended from the eighth grade to my senior year, especially the last two and a half years. I was bullied from eighth grade to the middle of tenth grade. But the bullies left and I began to turn my life around. That seventh grade teacher would have been surprised to see me playing for the school softball team, working on the school newspaper during my senior year and being elected student body president. By graduation, I was no longer frustrated by my autism and I went on to college in southern California.

One positive thing about my autism that started to develop early on was my visual memory. In second grade, my sisters discovered that I had memorized the names of all of the comic strips in the newspaper and their artists. My family and I went on a trip through the Midwest and someone gave me a placemat printed with all the states and their capitals. I soon had all of them memorized. Someone could give me a state and I could name the capital and *vice versa*. I began hoping that I could be on a television game show one day, a hope that I still carry with me.

That incident with *I Love Lucy* foretold things to come, and it wasn't until years later that I realized that I could use this skill to my advantage. In the last few years I have been building up an encyclopedic knowledge of television shows. I plan on being a writer for television when I graduate from college, and one of my professors told me that this ability would be helpful when I enter the industry. This is another way that I have managed to make my learning difference work in my favor.

There have been many negative comments expressed about autism, as if it's a curse. I don't feel cursed at all. Autism has given me an exciting and different way to view the world. Far from making my life hopeless, autism has not only led to my hopes of landing a job as a writer for TV drama, but it may help me if I find myself in front of the camera... as a game show contestant!

Brian Lafferty is a student at the University of California at Fullerton at work on a degree in radio, television, and film. He hopes to write television drama when he graduates.

Part IV
The Clouds Part

I Don't Understand

Michael Johnson

I don't understand
why some kids have autism
why those who can speak say mean things
why I can't sing when I would love to
But most of all
why life is unfair
why there are wars
why people I love move away
why life gets more complicated as I get older
What I understand most is
why I must keep trying
why math makes sense
why scientists ask questions to find answers
why love is the most important thing.

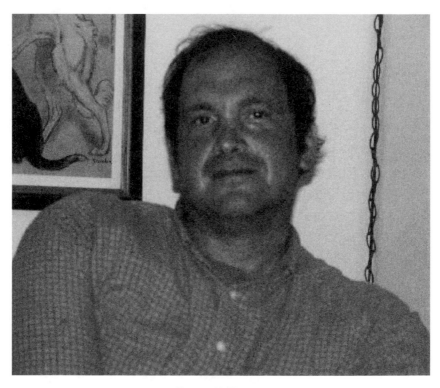

Perry Hoffman

Run Tiger Run!

Perry Hoffman

Autism found me on a hilly street corner in the Bronx during the summer of '63. It surrounded my body, scrambled my mind and silenced my voice. Mugged me in broad daylight in front of unsuspecting bystanders going about their daily routines. The assault isolated me, made me feel different and alone, as if I was placed in a bubble that consumed me whole.

That autumn, while millions were watching the exploits of Ben Casey, Andy Griffith and Fred Flintstone on television or listening to the Four Seasons and Leslie Gore on their transistor radios, the chains of autism tightened their grip on me. I spent my days wandering around classrooms, continuously humming T.V. theme songs and counting U.S. flags flying from apartment buildings. Teacher notes came home to mother. Men and women wearing white coats and Buddy Holly glasses popped open their folders and grilled me with questions. Wires were glued to my forehead. More tests, more doctors, more tears running down my mother's face.

After three years of tests, interviews and classroom pullouts, the doctors finally arrived at a conclusion. In a waiting room at a pediatrician's office in Brooklyn in 1966, my mother finally received the news.

"About your son, Mrs. Hoffman," the pediatrician said. "He has autism."

From then on, instead of walking four blocks to school, I rode a yellow bus that took me to a building three miles away. The chains of autism continued to tighten. Thoughts occurred to me over and over, uncontrollably. Flags, holidays, T.V. theme songs dominated my ride to school. If the thoughts became too intense, I would think about a commercial for Uniroyal tires that always came on during the evening news. It was a cartoon featuring a tiger running down a road, braving the elements. I would marvel at this tiger as he plowed through the toughest terrain. *Run tiger run! Harder! Faster! Forget about those children who laugh as I board the yellow bus. Keep going, tiger!*

Autumn 1967.

Year Two of Special Ed.

I am lying on a navy blue cot in the back of a fifth floor classroom. My teacher is at her desk, jotting a few notes on a pad. It is 1:30 in the afternoon, and I shun the idea of a nap. I thumb through a set of Golden Books. I use this time to navigate my imagination. I can go into space with the Gemini astronauts, enjoy an outdoor breakfast with Captain Kangaroo and friends, or think about the metallic-looking calendar stationed by the blackboard.

My five other classmates also try to exist in a system that has all but forgotten them. One is here because he is hyperactive, another is emotionally disturbed. One girl said she is here because she has an IQ of 81. I have been relatively quiet today, did not communicate with anyone except for a pair of boys in the bathroom, who made references to my classroom as "the faggot class."

I remain on my cot and do my utmost to ward off boredom, staring at the metallic calendar stationed near the blackboard. I fix my eyes on October 12th, marked with blue to denote Columbus Day. My mind is consumed with all thoughts Columbus, from the names of the three ships and his dealings with Queen Isabella to his landing on the Atlantic coast and exclaiming, "I am here! I discovered America!"

After nap time, the teacher starts her afternoon lesson. She asks me a series of questions that I don't comprehend; my answers are incoherent and disjointed. Teacher follows up with more questions. I blurt out something, but I don't know what. She grows frustrated. She describes me as being in outer space. I resume my thoughts about Columbus, amidst the roaring waves, on his knees, surrounded by the watercolor paint jars, the yellow clock with the big wheels, the wads of clay by the easel, and the Speak and Say game on the play station.

Sometimes, in desperation, my teacher will assign to me "cubby work," a portfolio of tasks and activities centered on linking and matching words, understanding concepts using fill-ins. I'll delve into the project for a few minutes, until my thoughts give way to parades, last night's television programs, animals, and holidays. Inevitably, my teacher's patience wears thin and I find myself back in pediatricians' and psychologists' offices doing an endless array of tasks and assignments. The clinics and centers see little progress in my efforts and commit me to Special Ed indefinitely.

In the meantime, I find comfort at home with my mother and my sister Toni and find added solace every evening when I watch television to keep abreast of the doings of my friend, the Uniroyal tiger. The tiger continues to run down the road. The mass of orange, black, red and white. His magnificent claws keep on course down the road.

Run tiger run! Harder! Faster! Keep going, tiger! He will be with me for a long time.

Autumn, 1972.

Third year of inclusion, six years after diagnosis.

Competent authorities discovered that I can speak in sentences, so they decided to send me to middle school. I am now separated from paint jars, yellow clocks with big wheels, and cubby work. Culture shock. Instructors ramble on about prepositional phrases, verb tenses, past participles, isosceles triangles, compounds and solids, the Treaty of Versailles, Romeo versus Tybalt. Everything remains a blur. Cannot break away from the chains of autism. At least I don't have to lie on a blue cot anymore.

I manage to hit it off with a couple of teachers. I don't engage in conversation with peers, though there are exceptions. When the substitute fills in for the regular teacher, a dozen or so classmates take their chairs and make their way towards me for a rap session. They ask me a lot of questions. I become the hit of the party. They ask how one distinguishes a queer person from a normal person. What constitutes a period and how does a girl deal with it? They throw a lot of terms around, mixing in such words as "pussy" and "dildo" with the usual references to faggot, spastic, and retarded. I make a trip to the guidance office and talk to the counselor. He takes a quick glance at my file and says there is little that he or the school can do.

I take brisk walks during lunch. Think about the old days. Think about the Uniroyal tiger. The mass of orange, black, red and white as he barrels towards his destination.

Run tiger run! Harder! Faster! Keep going, tiger! He will be with me for a long time.

Autumn 1978.

Second year of college, 12 years after diagnosis.

It is all a blur. All of it. I am miles away from being an academic man, intellectual man, *New York Times* man. I am autistic man. Adam Smith. Who was that? Describe the reconfiguration of Reconstruction in the Antebellum South. What? What would Kafka's take on Voltaire's *Candide* be? I have no clue. What about that German philosopher? I can't seem to come up with that name.

After 20-odd credits, it's sinking in: I am not cut out for college life. Discourse has vanished into thin air. Professors write commentary in the margins of my term papers such as, "Please explain," or "What are you trying to say?"

Oh, and the women. There's a pretty brunette, cute as a button, who sits right behind me in Film Studies 102. She chats with me every time I enter the auditorium. I can't come up with anything to say. Autism has stolen my voice. She takes out her phonebook and looks at me when classes end.

Meanwhile, letters from the university make their way into my mailbox. Words like probation, expulsion, and dismissal appear under the letterhead. I guess the college and I have to talk. I place the letters inside my bookbag and forget about them. What was I going to say? Maybe they can send me back to a special school.

Thoughts about Yankees/Red Sox, Christmas and the new Pope circulate in my mind. There is music in my head, selections from The Eagles, Fleetwood Mac and Billy Joel. Sometimes my thoughts are of things that happened to me twenty years ago, like looking at pink and green houses, replaying images over and over. I reminisce about the tiger in the Uniroyal commercial that ran down that rugged and slippery road. The brilliant hues of orange, red, black and white mix brilliantly as he runs.

Run tiger run! Faster! Harder! Keep going, tiger! He still is with me for a long time.

Winter 1985.

Five years since being removed from college, 19 years after diagnosis.

Following my college disgrace, I trade in my textbooks to become a shipping clerk for a prestigious jewelry firm, packing boxes for a living. Punch the clock and put my brain in the locker along with the jacket and the morning edition. For four years, nine months and twenty days I put precious stones, 14-carat gold chains and pendants into 8x14 cardboard boxes, stuff them with paper, put strips of tape on both sides and place the packages in a bin, ultimately rolling them down a conveyer belt. I apply for another position in the company that I know to be open, only to be told it isn't. Then, one day in February, the guys over in personnel call me on the carpet and say they no longer need my services.

After the layoff, I get hired to work part time in a school health program, where I administer hearing and vision examinations to children. Because I'm wet behind the ears, I ask my supervisor a lot of questions. She answered with things like, "You ask a lot of stupid questions, don't you?"; "You have a brain, don't you? Well, use it and think." One day I see her quietly leaning against the entrance to a school we are visiting, tears falling softly on her cheek. They always say that people in the spectrum are incapable of understanding feelings, but for some crazy reason, I can't help but feel sorry for her.

I ask my personal therapist what I should do about my autism. He responds, "There are things that every man should be able to deal with on his own. That is one of them." I think of things that brought me happiness as a child: staring at the pink and green houses in the old neighborhood, marveling over breakfast cereal boxes and the tiger from the Uniroyal commercial who ran down the road undaunted and determined, through all hazards and obstacles. The brilliant hues of orange, red, white and black, a magical kaleidoscope.

Run tiger run! Faster! Harder! Keep going, tiger! He will stay with me for a long time.

Autumn 1991.

Senior year in college, 25 years after diagnosis.

In the summer of 1986, I decide to give college another shot. By some miracle, I am accepted. Five years and 70-odd credits later, I am now within striking distance of graduating with a B.A. in English. Essays and research papers continue to elicit teacher criticism, but things appear to be finally coming into shape. Things don't seem to be as blurry as they once were. Sure, there are the occasional problems, but the victories seem to outnumber the defeats.

Along with the inroads made academically, there is some forward progress in social activity. There is the typical date, a group function or a picnic involving former coworkers. But all in all, euphoria is short-lived. The missed social cue, the lack of initiative, upends any momentum. Autism maintains its grip on me through these situations. I try to marshal all my energies to survive. Nevertheless, my family tells me that I have made great strides since I decided to return to school. I keep my focus and wait for that day in January when I graduate. I think of the perseverance of the tiger in that commercial that I first saw 24 years ago, who clawed and plowed his way through the rugged terrain.

Run tiger run! Harder! Faster! Keep going, tiger!

2007.

Five years after earning an M.A. in Education, 40 years after diagnosis.

Current vocation: teen counselor.

Today a 17-year-old young lady enters my office. She's just learned that she is pregnant. In a flash, her world is turned upside down. She worries about her college prospects, the reactions of her friends and parents, her boyfriend, the need to acquire services and entitlements, the rush to secure a good practitioner, and, most importantly, her future. In some bizarre way, I have gone full circle. Some 40-plus years ago, my mother was told the news that it was all over. She was told to prepare for a life of trial and hardship, for herself and the rest of her family.

As I prepare a bag of health literature and write a referral for my client to see the nurse, I can't help but see the parallels between my mother and this mother-to-be. At particular moments in their lives, both were told of the long odds they faced. Thankfully, my mother, my sisters and friends did not heed that dire prediction. It is through their efforts and love that I was able to pass through those obstacles.

I've just marked the 40th anniversary of my official diagnosis. I did not celebrate the occasion by recalling particular milestones. The events I have described are just intervals in anyone's life; the only difference is that I experienced them from an autistic person's perspective.

Forty years later, autism retains its tight grip on me. I wake up with autism, go to sleep with autism, eat lunch with autism, make a purchase at Macy's or Best Buy with autism, read books by Stephen King or Daniel Tammet, sit on the 40-yard line, enter a voting booth, see the 12 o'clock matinee, and go on a first date with autism. I was born with it. I will die with it. When I consciously realized that I was different on that Bronx street corner back in '63, I figured autism would be short-lived. Now I know that autism is forever.

Shortcomings and gifts are part of the autism package, and when life's little inconveniences and unfairness get just a little too unbearable, I find that there is a perfect way to escape all the insanity. I can go on YouTube and look for the Uniroyal tiger. And in an instant I am back in 1967 and I feel like I am watching the cartoon for the very first time. I am back in a very safe and comforting place, far away from the white rooms filled with lab technicians and doctors. I am back, glued to the screen, watching my friend run down that road. The brilliant hues of orange, black, red and white make up a magnificent tapestry. Poetry in motion. Using his sheer determination to claw and plow through all that terrain to get to his destination.

Run tiger run! Harder! Faster! Go tiger go!

Perry Hoffman has a master's degree in secondary education from Queens College of the City of New York and a Bachelor of Arts degree in English from Hunter College. He is a public health advisor and advocate for first-time teen mothers in the Nurse Family Partnership Program for the New York City Department of Health and Mental Hygiene, and he is a frequent presenter at regional conferences for autism and Asperger syndrome.

A Forever Mum

Christina England

I had completed my adoption application forms. On them, I specified, *"No autism."* Autism conjured up for me thoughts of rocking and screaming, of children who could not be loved. I was twenty-eight when I decided to adopt. I was single and working in a respite unit for disabled children, many of whom were waiting for adoptive parents to give them a chance. I watched with great sadness for years as they waited for their chance to join a "forever family." It seemed that their severe disabilities would keep them from adoption forever. Then I met my two boys. They would change my distorted preconceptions of autism and, more importantly, change my world forever.

During my time at the unit, I met a single lady who had adopted a girl of fourteen despite the child's severe disabilities. It was during my talks with her that I decided I also wanted to give a child a chance. I wanted to become a "Forever Mum." Four years later, after many assessments and rejections, I was introduced to Daniel, a blonde, blue-eyed four-year-old. His wobbly walk made me smile. I fell in love, probably for the first time. His disabilities were described as Global Developmental Delay with motor coordination problems. While completing the paperwork, I remember thinking, *well, that hides a multiplicity of sins.* How right I was.

A year later, Daniel was diagnosed with mild ataxic cerebral palsy, which explained the unsteady wide gait and clumsy actions. However, his real problem was not diagnosed at the time; it took eight years to get to the bottom of it. Daniel became aggressive, with no sense of danger. He would bite and kick. He was obsessive and compulsive, with no empathy for others. In his world, no one existed apart from him. He would also follow me everywhere. I put this down to the fact that he had been moved among foster parents five or six times. His main fear seemed to be sleeping alone. This worsened during the first year and he screamed all night, every night, telling me that monsters were trying to take him away from me. He could only be calmed if I took him to bed with me. Eventually, I bought a tent and put it next to my bed. Gradually, over the months, I moved it away little by little until he was outside my bedroom and in his own. Patience was the key and I was not one to give up.

Daniel continued on as a difficult, uncooperative child, almost impossible to look after. At one point my mother said to me, "He is impossible, why don't you give him up and take him back?" I said, "No Mum, I can't. I am his Forever Mum. Everyone gives up on him. There must be a way." One day shortly after this, Daniel came up to me and said, "Mum, when you want to throw me away like rubbish, like my other Mums, can you let me know first?" I said, "Dan, I will never do that, I am your Forever Mum and Forever Mums are forever."

When Daniel was nine I adopted my second son. Again I had stipulated on the adoption forms, "*No Autism.*" Nicholas was three and also diagnosed as developmentally delayed. Nick had no speech, had only just got onto his feet, and was still in nappies and not eating solids. He had been waiting for a family all his life and although I was desperate for a little girl, Nick won my heart with his jolly smile and cute looks.

Within months he was all over the place and on the go 24/7. He soon developed epilepsy and asthma and was continually ill. He would rock and flap and spin on the spot. As his speech developed he just repeated whatever was said around him. Over the next few years he began to demand that everything be in a particular order and would scream hysterically if anything was out of place. He was extremely hyperactive and always running away. I had to keep my eyes on him every second, as he had no awareness of danger at all.

Nick is very afraid of red, especially red food. He hates loud noises and getting wet, but he loves rubbing labels, silk and velvet. These textures can fascinate him for hours. When he was younger he liked opening gates, closing them, opening them, coming out and closing them again. A simple walk could take hours. Now he is a little better, if you can keep hold of him.

When Nick was seven and Dan was thirteen they were both assessed by an independent psychologist who found that Dan has Asperger syndrome, severe dyslexia and conduct disorder. Nick was diagnosed with ASD, dyspraxia, dyslexia and ADHD. So much for "*No autism.*"

That was eight years ago. My children have taught me that having autism is not a problem, but a challenge. Now 21, Dan swims for Great Britain in Disability Sport and his efforts have taken him all over the world. He is in college studying Arts and Media. Nick is 15 and he does struggle. He still flaps and rocks, he believes totally that he is a secret agent and that Dr. Who and the Daleks are real. He still runs away, likes order and is so literal he makes my head spin sometimes. Conversation in our house is almost impossible as no one understands anyone else, me less than anyone. But we understand love; there are masses and masses of it.

I consider myself lucky to have chosen two such lovely children, and being a Forever Mum is no problem. I have taught them both that *Forever Mums stay.* They have taught me not to run away from autism but to embrace it, because in this world, no one is perfect.

Born in London, Christina England's parents provided a foster home to many children for decades. It was because of her memories of childhood and her work in a respite unit that she decided to adopt. She hopes her experience will help others considering adoption to think about adopting a child with special needs. This story is dedicated to her two boys: some people make the world a special place by just being in it.

Just a Little Offbeat
Erin Vick

I stood there, knowing I was going to die. My face would turn red, it would start to burn, flames would erupt and poof, I'd be gone. My embarrassment would cause my spontaneous combustion. In the middle of Kmart.

"Mom, please, please make her take it off."

I pleaded with my mother for a third time as I followed behind the shopping cart she was pushing with *her* in it: the reason for my impending demise.

"I already told you no. She's not hurting anyone, she's content and I don't want to hear her scream if I try to make her take it off."

There my four-year-old autistic sister sat in the outfit she had been wearing everywhere for the past several months. Lace socks on her hands, a green and white striped ski cap on her head, and a wicker planter from one of my grandmother's potted plants on top of the ski cap. Imagine the looks we got.

So then I did what any ten-year-old would do: I pouted and prayed we wouldn't run into anyone from my school.

Growing up in a household with an autistic sister made for an interesting childhood. Autism affects thousands of people so I know I was not unique, but I didn't know anyone else going through what I was going through. No one I knew had a sibling who, when upset, would bang her head into the wall and feel no pain, who could spin in a circle for an hour and not be dizzy, who would always line up her toys in a specific order, an order that made sense to only her. No self-help books, no heartfelt anthologies to make me feel warm and fuzzy. I just had to muddle my way through it.

I honestly do not remember much else from when she was a baby. I was busy with my own seven-year-old life. I was completely unaware that my mom was noticing that something wasn't right with my sister. That she had started talking, gaining a few baby words, and then stopped. That she wouldn't make eye contact. That the only sound she ever made was da-da-da over and over again. I didn't know that life was about to change.

"Her brain is like a heart, and every once in a while it skips a beat."

That was how my mom explained Jamie's autism to me. That she was just a little offbeat from everyone else. I didn't know until I was older that when she was first diagnosed with autism, my parents were told that she would never talk, never learn how to do much of anything. She would basically be a bump on a log for the rest of her life.

I seriously don't know how I would react to that daunting news if I was a parent. I think most people would crumble. But my parents didn't. I'm sure there was some inner crumbling and internal screaming, but they didn't let that deter them. They researched autism, talked to people and put Jamie into behavioral therapy. To me, this meant that twice a week I got to go with my mom and sister and play Barbies with a college student named Debra who kept me busy while my sister was in her sessions. I had to sit on the sidelines while my sister got to ride horses as part of therapy.

I would like to say that I was a perfect angel during my teenage years, but that would be a big fat lie. I was rife with teenage angst and had a smart mouth that seemed to constantly get me in trouble. My parents were strict, not in a *Mommy Dearest* sort of way, but they had their rules, many of which I didn't agree with. In one of the more memorable fights with my mom, I uttered the words all kids have said and all parents have heard, "That's not fair!"

The response I received was, "Well, is it fair that you can go down the street and play with your friends and your sister can't? Or that you can go off to the movies with your friends and your sister more than likely never will?"

Whoa. Hold on there. The argument we were having had nothing to do with my sister. This was harsh and made an already angry teenager even angrier. All I could think of was that it wasn't my fault my sister would never do any of those things so don't put that on me. Looking back, I understand that I had pushed far beyond my mom's boiling point and she just vented her frustration, not at me but at our family's situation.

It was hard. We couldn't go many places because Jamie would refuse to leave the house. She would have the occasional screaming fit. Anytime we would go somewhere, we would have to cart huge bags of her toys to keep her occupied. Anytime we went out to eat, we had to make sure the restaurants served either cheeseburgers or grilled cheese sandwiches because she only eats a small variety of foods. It hurt that she was never invited to a birthday party. It hurt that I would never have a normal sister-sister relationship with her, that I would never be able to pass down my advice on makeup and clothes, would never share gossip about boys and friends. There would be no future holiday meals where my family and her family would get together and our kids would play.

She advanced far beyond what we had been told to expect. She learned to read and write, and was mainstreamed into many regular classes. She loves video games and has a deep fascination with anime, which for the life of me I don't understand. She talks, very loudly at times, and is sometimes hard to understand. I get frustrated with her; she could try the patience of a saint. We argue, like any normal pair of siblings.

Yeah, she's different, but she's my sister. She's the one who comes screaming into my room every Christmas morning, telling me Santa has come. She's the one who screamed the loudest when I graduated from college. She's the one who, if she feels I've slept in too late, will sneak into my room to see if I'm still alive. Weird I know, but it's her own way of showing that she cares. We will never have that normal sisterly relationship that I had once wanted, but the one we do have is not so bad.

Erin Vick lives in Houston, Texas, and graduated from Baylor University with a degree in forensic science. She is an avid reader and started writing stories not long after she learned the alphabet.

Our Village
Bev Schellenberg

An African proverb says, "It takes a village to raise a child," and our little village was terrified when my nephew Micah was diagnosed with autism at the age of two. It seems forever ago that my sister-in-law voiced her fears about her youngest son. And the rest of us in the family knew that she was right: something was terribly wrong.

Soon after Micah's birth we could see my tiny nephew's frustration, the pain of over-stimulation in a world of achingly brilliant lights, sounds, smells, tastes, and touch.

Although I'd been a teacher for several years, I didn't know what to do. I'd never taught an autistic child; I didn't know how to act around him. After I'd hugged the other family members he would stand, rocking from one foot to the other. Should I hug him? Would he let out his high-pitched scream, his body rigid? Once he began to slowly overcome the hurdle of language, I was at a loss again: when he repeated a TV commercial word for word, his face towards me, should I say anything? I didn't even know if he saw me.

Despite temper tantrums, toilet training an apparent impossibility and speech setbacks, Micah passed through each door of maturation with his family leading him through. When aspects of life became too difficult, his parents added members to their village: a speech therapist, a special needs daycare provider. And Micah taught us all what was right for him: for several years touch wasn't okay. Acknowledging his words was important. Allowing him to be himself was most important of all.

My daughter, Emma, was oblivious to her cousin's challenges. By the time she was walking and talking, visiting Micah was the highlight of her life and his as well. Although he was four years older, he played with the same toys as Emma, and he dealt with similar issues: fear of doctor visits, a need to have his daily routine explained.

However, it was a different situation when my son arrived. For some reason, Micah assumed a boy cousin would be born old enough to play with Star Wars figures. Micah thought that his newborn cousin should provide appropriate words for each Star Wars character as well as sounds and movements; sucking on them didn't count. His baby cousin's inability to even sit up or talk was unacceptable. "Jared's a bad boy. Jared's a bad boy," was how Micah summed up the problem.

It was Micah's mom who discovered a way to greatly reduce his frustration and to increase his coping skills. She began learning about autism the day Micah was diagnosed, and has never stopped. She is also an amazing cook, a natural at whipping together anything, be it a spaghetti dinner or a turkey dinner worthy of two pages in the *Saturday Evening Post.* Her research on autism led her to believe that a restricted diet sometimes improved an autistic child's ability to function. Despite the difficulties of getting a seven-year-old, even without autism, to eat anything different from the usual mac and cheese and hot dogs, she successfully removed wheat from his diet.

The results were not immediate. We wondered if it was worth the extra money and the time spent learning and creating new recipes. But it seemed to work: Micah went from parallel play to full interaction with his cousins within a month. When his mom did reintroduce wheat, he seemed to become highly agitated. That was the last of the wheat in Micah's diet. After a few months, Micah, like an older brother resigned to his position, showed Jared how to roll a ball, allowed him to watch computer games, and even explained the difference between a Storm Trooper and a Jedi Knight. When Micah learned to read, he read to Jared.

As the years went by I discussed Micah's autism with my children. They simply nodded. Later, after school one day, I brought the topic of Micah's autism up again in a conversation with my now seven-year-old daughter. She was having difficulty understanding an older student's unique behavior. "Why does he act different?" she asked.

"Perhaps he's autistic, like Micah, or he has challenges of a different kind."

"What do you mean, 'like Micah'?"

"Well, you know. Micah has autism."

"Yeah, so?"

"Well, he acts different sometimes, too."

"Oh. I never really noticed."

I was reminded of that conversation a few months later as our family sat again around my sister-in-law's table. Conversation predictably veered towards our children's experiences over the past weeks. "Micah's grown two clothing sizes in a matter of months. His pants were three inches too short for him, until I found some bigger ones," she said. She spooned out some more of her homemade cranberry sauce, and added, "He went to camp a couple of weeks ago."

"Where?" I asked.

She explained that he traveled on a bus to attend a camp for three days with his fellow grade six classmates and the grade seven classes from his school.

I looked at Micah. "How was it, Micah?" It was about this moment it dawned on me that Micah had gone without his parents, without his family, to a camp far, far away, and I hadn't heard anything about it before or during the event. It was a typical discussion of a boy's first trip to camp.

"Good. It was good," he said, between mouthfuls of roast beef, a newly acquired taste for him. "I wasn't able to brush my teeth, though. Not for the entire time."

"Why?" For a child with such a strong need for routine, this was peculiar.

"I never had two-and-a-half seconds. There was no time."

His mother told me the rest of the story later, as we were putting the food away. Micah was having so much fun he forgot to brush his teeth. The aide who traveled with Micah never actually said, "Micah, it's time to brush your teeth." The result? After the camping trip was over, Micah managed to survive the drive all the way back to school, but when he finally got into the family car and they started off, he couldn't take it anymore—he told his mom to stop the car. Then he rummaged through his bag for his neglected toothbrush, and brushed his teeth.

Micah stayed in a camp with his peers, in a cabin with his friends, in a world of archery, rock-climbing, swimming, crafts, and communal table dining. Did he act differently from the other children? Probably. He does have autism. But ultimately, as Micah has taught our family, and as my daughter so aptly said, "So?"

Bev Schellenberg is a freelance writer, writing instructor, high school educator, choral director, and parent. Her articles have appeared in anthologies and *The Globe* and *Mail*, and she writes for backofthebook.ca. She lives in the Pacific Northwest with her family and their vertically challenged miniature wiener dog, Cinnamon.

Work in Progress
Robin J. Silverman

Someone called today, out of the blue, to offer my daughter a job. Amazing. We turned down the offer; Lauren already has a job she loves. Truly amazing.

Why amazing? You have to know her job history.

Over the years, my husband and I have despaired that even with the help of a job coach, Lauren would ever be able to hang onto a job. We've had plenty of reason to doubt. I don't remember all the jobs, but a few stand out in my memory like scars on my psyche.

Lauren, 25, has Asperger syndrome and attention deficit disorder. She has multiple learning disabilities, impaired social skills and distractibility. Early on, Lauren worked in a church childcare program. It seemed like a good fit—not too demanding and run by kind people. Lauren likes children, has a lot in common with them. She played with the kids, helped feed them their snacks and did other small chores. The job went fairly well until one day when Lauren got angry with one of her charges for not getting up from his nap quickly enough and dumped him out of his cot onto the floor.

So much for childcare.

Then there was the packaging manufacturing company. The job, which involved assembling packaging, was too complicated for her, requiring multiple steps that Lauren couldn't master. Instead of placing her elsewhere, her job coach kept trying to make the work more manageable. With the best of intentions, the coach tried to force my square peg into this round hole until Lauren was so frustrated, she walked into a company bathroom and scribbled all over the walls with a permanent marker.

So much for manufacturing.

At this point, the people who ran the high school jobs program were running out of ideas for placements for Lauren. So we asked a friend of ours, the medical director of an assisted living facility who was serving as the interim director, if she might have a position. She hired Lauren to work in the supply room, where Lauren kept track of inventory and restocked shelves as needed. Part of her job was pushing a large cart around the facility, delivering medicine and other supplies to the medical staff and caretakers.

Lauren, who's very chatty, loved talking to the residents and staff, which made it difficult for her to stay on task. She also needed frequent reminders to be careful pushing the cart, which she tended to ram into things and people. But all in all, she did okay and the residents enjoyed having her around.

Unfortunately, the facility was embroiled in ugly politics. A permanent director came on board and started making staff changes, including replacing our friend the medical director. Once again, we saw handwriting on the wall, but this time it wasn't Lauren's. The new administration let Lauren go, citing budget cuts. As though 20 hours a week at minimum wage was going to break the institution.

So much for politics.

Staff changes put the kibosh on Lauren's next job, as well. A kind and grandmotherly store manager hired Lauren and worked alongside her to help her learn the job. She taught Lauren how to stock shelves, clean windows, take out trash and help customers find what they were looking for. But when the manager transferred to another store, no one else was willing to give Lauren the supervision she needed to do a good job.

Instead of firing her, the new manager kept cutting her hours until Lauren was working only a few hours a week. The khaki pants she had to buy to wear to work cost more than she was making. At that point, we had her quit while her job coach looked for a more suitable placement. Ironically, Lauren had been one of the most reliable workers at that store; unlike much of the staff, she showed up when she was assigned and did the job she was given.

So much for retail.

Next came a volunteer stint at an animal shelter, where Lauren was told she had a chance of being hired if she did well. She loved working with animals so much that she didn't mind cleaning up after them or getting scratched, or even bitten. But speed seemed to be the main job requirement. No matter how hard she tried, Lauren never could clean the cages fast enough to satisfy her supervisor. I found it perplexing that the supervisor, who devotes her life to the care of abandoned animals, had so little compassion for a human in need. When Lauren's trial period was over, she wasn't invited to join the staff.

So much for volunteerism.

At my hair stylist's suggestion, I recently caught an episode of the TV reality show *America's Next Top Model*. James wanted me to see it because of Heather, a contender with Asperger syndrome, who had made it to the top five. A stunning, photogenic 21-year-old, Heather bungled the challenges. The contenders were given a time limit to get to several "go-sees," appointments with fashion designers. Heather got lost (did I mention they were in Shanghai?), so she made it to only one of her appointments, where the designer criticized her for not making eye contact while she modeled the clothes. Then she had difficulty finding her car, and was 40 minutes late completing the challenge. She was eliminated from the competition.

Watching Heather, I couldn't help but think about Lauren, about the times our daughter has lost out because of her disability, about the expectation that she learn to do things her disability makes impossible for her. Even well-meaning sorts—those who work with people with disabilities—expect Lauren to overcome her impulsivity, her social awkwardness, her lack of attention.

As I watched Heather frantically trying to read a Chinese map, I thought of how well she photographed and how beautifully she showed off the clothes, presumably the main requirements of modeling. So why couldn't she have an assistant to help her organize and get to appointments on time? I realize Heather was in a competition, but her experience wasn't so different from everyday life. Many people with disabilities could do bang-up jobs if only they had the support systems they needed. To thrive in a job, Lauren, like others with disabilities, needs close supervision and a commitment from those in charge to work with her abilities.

We got lucky with Lauren's latest job. The stars aligned just right: she has a job coach who knows how to develop jobs for people with disabilities, work she loves, and a supervisor who gives her the direction she needs to do the job well. We once worried if Lauren could handle working 15 hours a week. She now works 30.

Lauren plays with dogs at a PetSmart Doggie Day Camp. She also cleans up their messes, walks them and gives them their treats. She's been bitten and scratched and peed on, and she doesn't mind a bit.

Lauren's offer of another job, one she can afford to turn down, is gravy. We still worry that her supervisor will leave or that something else will change. But for now, we're thrilled.

Every afternoon, when my phone rings at 4:15, I know it's Lauren, calling to give me the doggie report. "Vito was there today," she says of one of her regulars, a pug. "And I got to give him his ice cream."

Robin J. Silverman is a freelance writer whose most recent work has focused on health issues. A frequent contributor to MayoClinic.com, she has also worked as a magazine and book editor. As a reporter, she wrote for *United Press International*, the *St. Louis Post-Dispatch*, *Communication World*, and the *Kansas City Business Journal*.

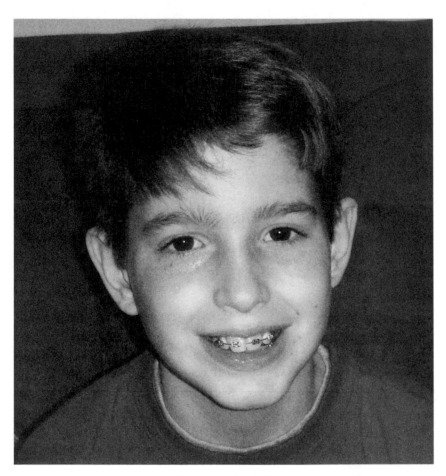

Zachary Mandel

I'm Sad, Too

Lee Mandel

"Why are you crying?" he asked with his usual blank stare. "Are you hurt?"

How could I explain death to a person who does not comprehend the feelings and emotions felt by other people? Of the many aspects of autism, the lack of empathy has been the hardest for me to accept. I looked at my eight-year-old son, Zachary, and took a moment to collect my thoughts. How would I explain it so he could understand? I know it isn't his fault, that he's disconnected, and I know it isn't my fault that I can't just hold him in my arms and transfer the knowledge and understanding I possess through kisses, but it is still very frustrating.

"Zachary," I started slowly, making sure to look him in the eyes in order to connect with him, "Grandpa died this morning." I knew that a straightforward approach always worked best with him. He didn't understand metaphors or hints, and couldn't gain perspective from observation. I sat across from him and waited for a response. I tried to read him and anticipate what he might say. "Do you know what that means?" This was his first experience with losing a loved one, other than the passing of our cat two years before.

"Yes. I'm not going to see Grandpa anymore." I felt my heart sink and the warm tracks of my tears as they streamed down my face.

His words were a harsh reality. I wouldn't see my father again either. But for Zachary it was more than that. My father had a deep connection with him, maybe the only emotional connection Zachary had ever had. They had been best friends. They saw each other every day, including weekends. They understood each other without the use of words. Their acceptance of one another's "quirks" was unconditional and admirable. Why would *this* have to be Zachary's first experience with death?

Although words usually come to me quite easily, I was at a loss. I sat on his bed, careful not to touch him, because he needs to grant permission first. I didn't want to be rejected. I wrestled with the new pain of losing a parent, while trying to keep a brave face and analyzing how Zachary was formulating his own definition of death.

We sat for a few moments in silence. Then he asked, "Where did he go? Is he with Cleo (our departed cat)?" This thought process wasn't what I was expecting, but I attempted to explain as best I could about the soul leaving the body and going to Heaven.

"There's two of him?" he continued. I made up a story about God placing a puzzle piece inside everyone's heart when they are born and needing to retrieve it at the end of that person's life, and that is when the body is no longer needed, just the puzzle piece. I continued by explaining the burial process and how it helps those of us still here to say "goodbye." I thought he would be frustrated with this explanation and lose control, but he remained quiet and unemotional.

Several more moments passed without inquiry. "Is there anything else you want to know about right now?" I asked.

"No."

"Alright, well, if you want to talk, or have any questions, you know you can come to me or Daddy, okay?"

"Yes." Without knowing what else to say, I left him, ready to drop whatever I was doing should he come to ask more questions.

On the day of the funeral I laid out the itinerary of events for Zachary, as must be done daily, especially with a new activity.

"Are you still sad?" he asked.

"Yes," I answered. "I think I will be sad for a long time. I'm going to miss Grandpa."

He collected a handful of trains, as he always does before leaving the house, and we began the longest and most difficult day of my life. Zachary sat at my side, unaffected, watching the parade of people come over to my mother and me to offer their condolences. He never made a sound and he didn't look at anyone. He kept his gaze focused on the tweed carpet in the funeral parlor.

As I watched my father's body being lowered into the ground, I could not hold my composure any longer. Between sobs, I felt a small hand tapping at the base of my back. I looked down to see Zachary standing beside me. "Don't be sad, Mommy. Grandpa is in Heaven now. He can still see us. We can't talk to him, but we can think about him all of the time even though we can't see him anymore." I realized in that moment that my son was exhibiting empathy and that *he* was consoling *me*. And then he said it: "I'm sad, too."

He wrapped his arms around my waist and gave me a big hug. It was amazing how in this time of loss, I experienced a gain—of hope for my son.

Every now and then Zachary and I sit and talk, and remember the many wonderful things we miss about my father, his best friend. At the end of our session, I am usually tearful. Zachary always puts his arms around me and says, "I miss him. I'm sad, too." Then we hug.

When the author is not reading or writing, she spends time with her husband, her two sons, who are both on the spectrum, two hyper dogs, and two very sleepy hamsters.

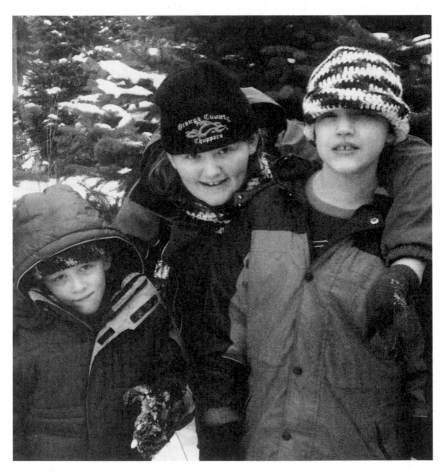

Bobby, Kathleen, and Billy Buick

My Special Brothers
Kathleen Buick

Some people like to write about themselves, but not me. I like to write about my brothers and what makes them special. My brother Billy is 8 and likes "goose bump" movies, taking baths, shopping and fashion. He loves summer so he can play in the water and jump on the trampoline. He gets very nervous during thunderstorms and likes to hang out with me and listen to stories. My other brother Bobby is 4 and likes cars, Daddy's tools, dinosaurs, Lego, trains and messing up the house. Bobby has lots of energy and loves to laugh, be silly and get into trouble. My brothers are the coolest brothers, even though they get on my nerves and can be really annoying at times. I am their big sister, so I guess that's to be expected, and I love them for it.

My brothers are loving and kind and thoughtful not only to me but to everyone around them. They teach me new things every day and I have become such a good person because of who they are. In my family, we see people for their abilities and what they have to offer. We don't put labels on them because of a medical diagnosis. We give people a chance by getting to know them for who they are. To me, my family is just like any other family: we love each other, we respect each other and we help each other.

So what is so special about my brothers? They probably sound just like any other brothers, except they have autism. You couldn't tell that from hearing about them and who they are and what they are like. In fact, you can't even tell they have autism from looking at them. They look like anyone else you see at the park or the store, except that they act somewhat differently from most. Even though they have autism, they both are like any other brothers: they make messes and make me mad and like to play with things that don't belong to them. But they are special because they have helped open people's eyes. My cousins, my aunts, my uncles, my grandparents, my friends and anyone else we know have a better understanding of people with disabilities from knowing my brothers and have learned to accept them for their abilities, not their disabilities. Their laughter, their smiles, their spirit reach out and touch people's hearts. You can't help but like my brothers once you take the time to get to know them.

My brothers have given me so much, so I give back to them by trying to be a good sister. I like to take Billy outside and teach him how to cross the street by looking both ways. I take him to my friend Mandy's house and he gets to play with her and her two sisters. They have also been touched by Billy's charm, and they ask him back time and time again. This is great, because Billy does not know many kids in our neighborhood, since he goes to a school that is far from our house. Someday, when Bobby is older, I hope to do the same for him.

I think it's the coolest thing to have brothers with autism. Anyone can learn a lot from them; I have. You can learn kindness and respect towards others who may have a disability or might be different from you. If you take the time to get to know someone for who they are, you might find out that person is special for more reasons than just their wheelchair, their braces, their glasses or the color of their skin. It is when you don't take the time and you let differences get in the way that you miss out on some of the best people you will ever know.

Everyone wants to be treated the same and have the same chances as everyone else. I think, *Why not, let it be so*! Reach out to others, help one another and make the world a better place. You will feel great and be a better person and make a new friend in the process. Who knows, it may even be my brother!

———————————

Kathleen Buick is a thirteen-year-old 7th grader from Rochester, New York. Her essay, *My Special Brothers,* won third prize in her middle school essay writing contest.

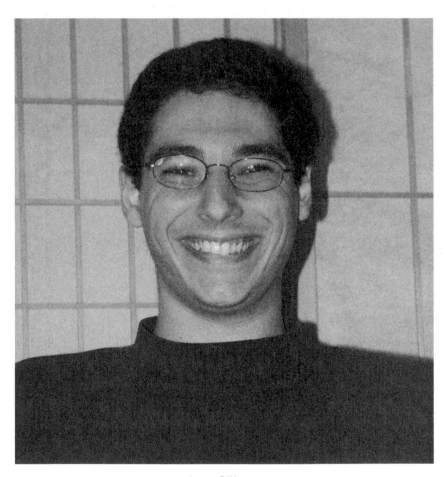

Aron Silberg

Aron's Bar Mitzvah

Barbara Silberg

Let me assure you that it is perfectly understandable if you laugh out loud at what I write here. To be honest, I tend to think my son's Bar Mitzvah was one of the funniest I've ever attended. Of course my handsome son, Aron—an extroverted, high-functioning autistic young man—would be the first to tell you that how he acted at his Bar Mitzvah, at age thirteen, was inappropriate. At twenty-one years of age, he knows that—now.

Looking back on it, we were very lucky. After all, before 1980 many special-needs children in the United States had neither gotten formal religious training nor undergone the rite of Bar Mitzvah. By the time Aron was ready to go to religious school, however, our Jewish Federation (at the urging of my uncle, Harold Reingold, the Director of Jewish Education at one of the largest synagogues in Houston) had been convinced to establish a special education Sunday school class for elementary children of various ages and handicaps.

Thus, when Aron reached first grade—a mere year after the class had been established—we enrolled him in the special-ed Sunday school class. He attended this special class until fifth grade. At age ten, when he was mainstreamed into a regular classroom, we placed Aron into regular Hebrew school at our synagogue. He thrived there, quickly learning more Hebrew vocabulary and more about Jewish customs. Once we got him into the habit of going to the children's services on Saturday mornings, my son swiftly picked up the prayers he needed to be able to conduct services.

When Aron turned twelve, to ensure that he would be ready for his Bar Mitzvah, we consulted the congregation's cantor. After speaking with the young clergyman—explaining to him some of the behavioral pitfalls Aron had faced and was still dealing with— and allowing for the fact that Aron's behavior was rather unpredictable at times, we agreed that an abbreviated, late Saturday night service (instead of a regular Friday night and/or Saturday morning service) would be better.

Soon Aron began studying his Torah portion (the Torah being the parchment scrolls containing the first five books of Moses) and his Haftorah portions (a selection from other books of the Bible). And while the boy diligently listened to the tapes of chanted Hebrew the cantor had given him to study, Aron's anxious parents dealt with all the other details: writing and printing invitations, arranging entertainment for his party, obtaining supplies, doing all the baking for the party and his reception at the synagogue, etc. The Thursday before the big day, Aron and the synagogue's new rabbi staged a brief rehearsal in the chapel. Afterwards—procrastinating as usual—with less than two days to spare, Aron prepared his Bar Mitzvah speech.

Finally came the momentous day.

Although Aron is now a lean and rangy six-footer, at the time of his Bar Mitzvah—poised for a coming growth spurt—he was a bit on the chunky side. He was not at all self-conscious, however. With many of his dark curls neatly hidden beneath a new blue yarmulke (skullcap), dressed in his new navy suit and a new blue tie, Aron was full of the pride of accomplishment even before the fact. His quick smile was unusually brilliant on the day of his Bar Mitzvah. He knew he was going to do well and was not even a little nervous.

Tradition in our synagogue has the child's family sit in the front pews. This serves to direct all the attention to the Bar Mitzvah boy (or Bat Mitzvah girl) on the podium and emphasizes the fact that these children are henceforth to be considered as adults in the religious community. Finding our seats on the first row, my husband Robert and I watched Aron mount the stairs.

Before any prayers began, my husband and I were called up to formally present Aron with his tallit—in this case, a traditional white prayer shawl with blue borders. After we returned to our seats, as Aron led the opening prayers, he did not notice his new tallit slipping down his shoulders. Fortunately, the new rabbi caught it just before it hit the floor, nonchalantly sliding it back across Aron's shoulders where it belonged.

Oblivious to the fact that any of our guests might have been embarrassed by his pointing out their late arrival, while continuing to chant the prayers Aron waved (discreetly, he thought) in greeting to friends and relatives as they filtered into the sanctuary. Aron likes doing things very quickly. Singing not being an exception, he ran through the prayers very rapidly, though accurately. As star of the show, not hindered by even a hint of stage fright, Aron was in his element. And since the service was a very short one anyway, we got to the Torah reading about seven minutes into the service.

Before this portion of the service begins, the rabbi traditionally hands the heavy Torah scrolls to the Bar Mitzvah boy. The boy, then, has the honor of carrying the precious scrolls as he leads a ceremonial parade around the chapel. Normally this is a decorous procession down the few stairs of the pulpit stage and into the congregation, accompanied by a dignified, stately tune. But when the rabbi placed the Torah into Aron's arms, the boy bolted down the stage's three stairs—as if a fire alarm had sounded in his head. I never thought of this portion of the service as an extreme sport before, but Aron seemed to.

Frankly, I was concerned he'd break his neck, dropping the Torah in the process. When he did neither I began to giggle, relieved. Of course, as the mother of the Bar Mitzvah celebrant, I felt it necessary to try to remain appropriately dignified. I did manage to smother my laughter, but tears gathered in my eyes with the effort. My shoulders were shaking so hard that anyone seeing me from the back must have thought I was sobbing.

In the meantime, because Aron was meeting and greeting those he knew as if he were a politician up for re-election, the rabbi and cantor were able to catch up to him. Thank heavens, one or both of them was able to convince Aron to return to the podium at a more ceremonious pace.

Aron stepped up to the Torah like a pro. Using his clear, strong, melodious voice, he chanted the *trop* (Hebrew musical notations) almost effortlessly. Effortlessly, that is, until he announced— loudly, of course—that he'd lost his place. With the able help of the cantor and rabbi, Aron quickly found his place again, continuing flawlessly with his Haftorah afterwards.

I couldn't hear Aron's speech for my nervousness for him. His words were simply a blur. The congregation seemed to enjoy it, however—laughing at whatever my clever son said.

When Aron ended his speech, the congregation tossed soft, pastel-colored jelly candies at him. He managed to catch many of the candies, gleefully throwing most back. For a few minutes, it looked like a scene from a Mardi Gras parade.

Even so, he did manage to scarf down at least one of the candies before proceeding with the service. Of course, when Robert and I heard Aron's protest of: "Oh man!" everyone knew that he was unhappy about the delay in eating the rest.

The second Torah procession, done before returning the scrolls to their resting place in the Ark, proceeded at the proper pace—with no sprinting involved.

After the Torah was stored away, Aron joined the rabbi at the microphone. Having blessed our young man, the rabbi presented Aron with a few gifts from the congregation. Now, while "normal" kids are happy to just stand there and—at most—nod, Aron has never been happy to just stand or just listen. So when the rabbi, pleased with Aron's accomplishments as we all were, complimented him on a job well done, Aron replied with an overloud but polite, "Thank you."

And though Aron's behavior thus far should have alerted the rabbi that Aron wasn't about to behave normally, the man didn't seem to have a clue. Laying his hand on Aron's shoulder, the new rabbi teased my boy: "I'm sure we can count on you to read another Torah portion, in three weeks." With every thought reflected on Aron's face, I could see him calculating how much more preparation time he'd need in order to learn a new portion. Sheer panic skated across his face, and with a vigorous shake of his head and a more emphatic, "Uh-Uh!" Aron made it plain that his momma hadn't raised a fool. He was not about to "volunteer" for such an honor, not with only three weeks to prepare.

It was time, then, for his parents to bless the Bar Mitzvah boy. Even as my husband, Robert, and I mounted the stairs and stepped to the podium, Aron—aware of my tendency towards stage fright—sought to reassure me. As he strode across the stage to join us, I'm convinced that everyone in the synagogue plainly heard his stage whisper: "Calm down, Mommy, calm down. It's okay, it's okay." I got through the blessing without even a hint of fear. I was too preoccupied trying not to laugh at my son's encouragement. And after all, who could be frightened with such a sweet son behind them?

And as night darkened the bright stained glass windows, we began the *Havdalah* service to bid the Sabbath goodbye. With the overhead lights dimmed, the braided blue and white *Havdalah* candle was lit. In the candlelight, as he began to sing the short prayers,

Aron's face beamed with satisfaction. Unfortunately, he also began to wave his hands up and down. (Apparently Aron had forgotten—or was simply ignoring—my earlier admonition *not* to pretend he was a choral director.)

To top things off, when the spice box was passed under his nose, Aron screwed up his face like he'd just been exposed to a plateful of sauerkraut. Acting as if he had never come near a spice box before, he asked indignantly, "What's that?" At the reception at the synagogue, Aron piled his plate high with cookies and sweets, happily accepting praise from one and all. Unfortunately, instead of nodding, he thanked them when his mouth was full—as usual.

Aron's Bar Mitzvah proved to be a joyous celebration. And, well... Aron was just being Aron.

Barbara Silberg is a writer who specializes in humorous verse, short stories, and ad copy. She lives in Houston with her husband, photographer Robert, their son, Aron, and the requisite cat.

A Strong Family Because of Fragile X

Dorothy Dillard

Cole is my stepson, and he has Fragile X syndrome. He came into my life when he was eight months old. He is now 10. His mother had to consult numerous pediatricians before a medical professional agreed to genetic testing. This resistance came despite a family history that included a nephew with Fragile X. It was not the medical professionals who came around first. It was Cole's childcare provider who began to affirm his mother's concerns, and eventually they were able to have him assessed through a child development program. That assessment opened the door to medical and educational interventions.

Cole has a rather severe case of Fragile X. He is ten but does not speak. But he knows exactly what is going on. He also knows exactly what he wants and communicates that clearly. His motor skills are underdeveloped. If he runs, it looks much more like a modern dance performance than running. He is just now using the bathroom on his own.

Cole enjoys people. Most of the time, he wants to be included. He loves to read and go to the park and be tickled and cuddled. Cole loves water. When he was a toddler I would cover the kitchen floor with towels, fill several large bowls with water and give him bathtub toys. Cole would spend hours splashing the toys into the pots and bowls. We recently went through a stage where the only place Cole was happy was in the bathtub.

Cole has an incredible sense of humor. His sisters ask him yes/no questions and he either nods or shakes his head. They ask him things like, "Is there a hippopotamus in your class?" Cole smiles and his big green eyes shine with that knowing look that he is about to fool you. And then he will nod his head and laugh with glee.

We embrace those moments because the challenges of Fragile X are immense at times. There are the minor things, like the repetition, that can be intriguing in some ways and annoying in others. Cole can rewind a video to the exact word in the middle of a sentence and replay a phrase repetitively, with truly impressive precision. Then, the half sentence repeated at full blast can test the patience of a saint.

Many weekends when Cole is at our home, we are "grounded." Social events are out of the question. Family activities are limited. When he is in a good place, Cole will enjoy the park. He loves the zoo. But any activities that do not involve animals or water and involve people are not likely to happen when Cole is with us. Cole's reaction to people and situations is unpredictable. We can all pack up, go to a park and be happily enjoying our outing when Cole gets freaked out. He will start to scream and physically freeze. He is getting too big for me to pick up, and trying to get him to move can be nearly impossible. Medication can be helpful. But on many occasions it has no effect.

Cole shuts out what he doesn't want to deal with by wringing his hands and screaming. Odd things set him off. My father. Books and DVDs neatly on the shelves (he must have all the books and DVDs spread across the floor). Brushing his teeth. The buzz of florescent lights. The hum of the refrigerators in the grocery store.

Cole can also get overexcited. The computer is his portal to thrill-ville. Cole, like many autistic kids, is a whiz on the computer. He can access things that I never knew existed. His speed coupled with his impatience, though, is problematic in cyberspace. In less than two minutes he has been known to open five start pages and 21 versions of a game. Next thing we know the house is rocking, literally, with the sound of the music of a computer game. Cole insists on having the sound off or at full blast; there is nothing in between for him.

Sleep, or more accurately, the lack thereof, is our greatest challenge. From the start, Cole has had trouble sleeping. My only clear memory of Cole as an infant is of holding him and rocking him for hours to the same CD. Fortunately, I loved the CD and still do. Several songs will always bring tears to my eyes because of the bittersweet experience of Fragile X.

Cole has well-honed manipulation skills, and he is very certain about where and with whom he wants to sleep. He can become physical if he does not get what he wants. As he gets bigger and stronger, battling with him physically is not an option. There is also the risk that he will freak out. At that point, even calming medications are not effective. The fear of Cole hurting himself or someone else lurks in every interaction that involves him doing or going somewhere he doesn't want to do or go. Most of the time, he is responsive to firm words and direction.

But there are a few situations in which he chooses to fight. At our home, the trigger is sleep. The sleep issue has become paramount. We are in the process of having Cole observed at a sleep clinic. We may not be able to complete the test. Cole's anxiety in medical settings has been so severe in a number of instances that the tests could not be completed. My husband and I are taking the lead on this one and, as his mother reminds us, we have no idea what we are getting into. This is the reality of Fragile X; we never know what Cole's reaction to things will be. We are meeting some resistance from the medical profession. Interventions and medications with unknown effects are being offered. Again, we are all trying to balance what is best for Cole and what is best for two different families. We tread lightly and always flexibly. We will find some compromise that works for all of us. And, again, we will be faced with another challenge. No different from raising any other child. Just much more complicated.

Fragile X kids have trouble regulating stimuli. Everything comes rushing in as top priority. Cole, like many other Fragile X kids, has learned some defenses. Low level squealing, covering his ears, turning the sound of computers and TVs either full blast or off are ways Cole tries to regulate the stimuli. I worry sometimes that our home is too much for Cole. It is far from a low stimuli environment. Here, Cole lives with three very verbal and very active sisters. There are numerous televisions, stereos and computers screaming for his attention. Dinner is a three-ring circus whether Cole is with us or not.

But every time Cole enters our home, he lets us know that he loves it here. He comes in and touches each of his sisters on the head and gives a giggle of glee. And I know that he is important to the girls because he can't leave without being escorted to his mother's car by all three of his sisters and covered with hugs and kisses. I have watched each of the girls go through a procession of stages in understanding and accepting Cole. As infants and toddlers, they saw his bouncing and screaming as their own personal entertainment. The two older girls have been through a stage of irritation and annoyance. Cole's lack of boundaries, which includes sitting on his sisters, changing the television station, eating food off their plates and taking books and toys, is far from entertaining.

Over the past year his older sister, who is seven, moved on to a better understanding and even interest in Fragile X. Her patience has grown and typically she tries to help Cole. She has learned to speak firmly but lovingly to him and to expect that he will be back in her space sooner than later. She has learned to converse with him and loves to ask him questions. She reads to him and helps him with puzzles. She doesn't moan when she realizes that Cole is coming for the weekend. In fact, she quickly and happily adjusts her schedule and expectations.

Our family has grown immensely stronger because of Cole. Cole reminds us of the fundamental truths necessary for happy families: spend time together; don't over-schedule activities; be flexible; be aware of what others need and where they are emotionally; hug a lot; say "I love you" even if you don't get a response; laugh together. Cole helps us keep it simple. Cole reminds us what is important in parenting: give your kids the space to define their worlds and make their own decisions as age appropriate. Listen to them no matter how they are communicating their needs and wants and feelings.

We have all learned patience and sharing beyond the typical lessons. We have all learned to adjust quickly, to be flexible, to put others first. To laugh. We have learned that our needs are frequently wants and that in the face of the physical and emotional pain of another we can let them go. We have learned to communicate in alternative ways, to listen with our hearts and our eyes, not just our ears. To appreciate the gifts we are given and the gifts others have.

Every night when I kiss my children, including Cole, good night, I tell them that they are beautiful, precious and perfect. And, no matter what else is happening or has happened or will happen, Cole has made our family more beautiful, precious and perfect than any of us could imagine. We are a stronger family because of Fragile X. Now that Cole is making progress, his maternal grandfather says with relief that he is finally "getting it." My guess is that *we* are finally "getting it."

Dorothy Dillard is the mother of three, stepmother of three more, and wife of one. She writes and teaches in Newark, Delaware.

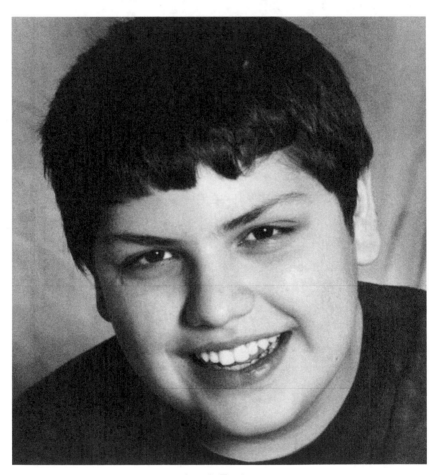

Jacob Tucker

What My Son Has Taught Me

Sherri Tucker

When my son was diagnosed with autism, a million thoughts went through my head. Had all of my dreams been erased? I felt as though my little boy would never lead a normal life and that nothing good would ever come of his autism. But that was eleven years ago. In those eleven years I have learned many valuable lessons from my son. Here are a few.

My son has taught me compassion. I will never again look at a child having a meltdown in the store and think that he needs a good spanking or that he has a bad mother. Instead, I will look into her weary eyes and try to convey my understanding.

My son has taught me honesty. He never sees a reason to lie. He is probably right. He will never break anyone's heart, steal from another the things that they have worked so hard for, or get something that he doesn't deserve. He won't lie to protect himself from punishment or to get out of something. He will accept the consequences of his actions because he simply doesn't see any other way to live. Truthful is the only way to be; I have learned this from my son.

My son has taught me tenacity. So many days I would like to just go back to the way my life used to be. With no need to research, advocate, call, write, get to know my legislators, get to know my school administrators, or fight one more battle. But if I don't, who will? Who will be the person that makes sure he lives up to his fullest potential, if I don't? My son has taught me never to quit.

My son has taught me to be supportive. Before he was born I was happy keeping my house spotless, my garden weedless, my life simple. Because of him I have learned the value of giving and receiving. I have met wonderful people and I thank God every day that He brought us together. I constantly hear that God doesn't give us more than we can bear. I believe that this time, He did. But He also gave us each other, knowing that we would help each other get through this.

My son has taught me to be assertive. I always believed that the experts knew everything and that we should blindly place our faith in them. I now know this is simply not true, and that without questions there can never be any real answers.

My son has taught me charity. He is willing to give anything that he has to someone who has less. He would give his most prized possession to another child. He would move a homeless person into our home. He would give his food to a hungry person. My son has shown me how selfish I can be and what the true meaning of a giving heart is.

My son has taught me love. He loves with no conditions. In his eyes, I am the most beautiful woman in the world. In his eyes, I am the most intelligent person on the planet. In his heart, I am the best Mommy that God ever created. Our lives are not what we had expected them to be. He will never be the President of the United States. He will never run a Fortune 500 company. He will never be a lawyer or a doctor. In truth, I have no idea what his future holds. But at night, when I lie down beside him and look into that angelic face, I can't imagine him any other way.

Sherri Tucker is the mother of three beautiful children, the co-founder of the Lee's Summit Autism Support Group, and a member of the Missouri Department of Elementary and Secondary Education Special Education Advisory Panel.

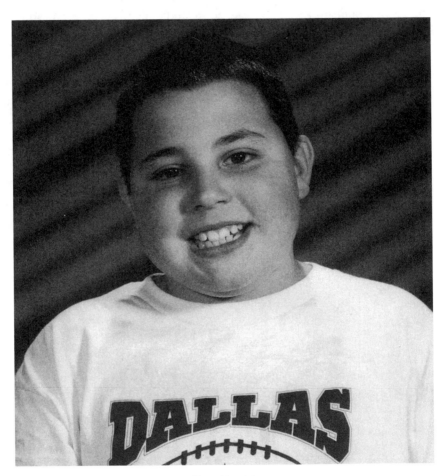

Dax Neeld

Life with Dax

Derek Neeld

My ten-year-old son Dax was diagnosed with autism at the age of four, and life with him has been an adventure. Dax was two when he started making "The Line" each night before bed. Dax had an enormous collection of Matchbox cars and trucks. He loved this collection and played with it all over the house and yard. Before bedtime, he would take this collection and make a very straight and ordered line of certain cars and trucks placed end to end. Everything in The Line had a specific place. Though Dax had dozens of cars and trucks in his collection, he always knew if one was out of place or, worse, missing. And since he played with them constantly, both inside and outside the house, it was a rare night when at least one or two weren't missing.

A missing car or truck meant a furious tantrum until it was found and properly placed in The Line. Dax was completely nonverbal at this time, so if a car or truck were missing, he couldn't tell us which it was. To make matters worse, there were cars and trucks in the collection that didn't make it into The Line on occasion and the composition of The Line varied from week to week. We'd go through the process of searching high and low for the missing car or truck, bringing those we found to Dax for inspection, hoping we had found the right one. Most often we hadn't and the search continued. This could take hours. If The Line wasn't complete, no one would get any sleep.

The Line lasted about a year. I wish I could say why Dax quit making it or that my wife Crystal or I did something that caused him to give it up, but I can't. Dax either outgrew The Line or simply got tired of it. We weren't sad to see it go.

Dax was three when he decided to be a dog. We had three dogs kept in the backyard and these were Dax's best friends. One morning after breakfast, Dax went outside to play with them. When Crystal looked outside to check on him a few minutes later, he was gone. She called me and together we searched the backyard but found nothing except his discarded clothes. We weren't concerned at first: not answering our calls wasn't unusual and taking off his clothes was nothing new, either. However, we began to worry after searching for him without success.

We were close to panic when Dax finally showed himself. Completely naked, he came crawling out from underneath the house. In his mouth he held an old squeak toy we had bought for the dogs. Crystal and I were both too shocked to do anything other than laugh. We tried to grab him, but he took off back under the house and sat near the opening, just out of arm's reach. We tried pretending to walk off, and when Dax poked his head through the opening, we'd try to rush over and grab him. We were always too slow. Finally, Crystal had an idea. She went into the house and returned a few seconds later with a box of doggie treats. Waving a treat in front of the opening, she was able to coax Dax out just enough for me to grab him. He growled and barked but I was able to drag him out.

That was the first time Dax decided he was a dog, but not the last. For the next year he sometimes urinated outside like a dog, leg hiked and all, and licked people on the face when he was happy. Once, he even tried to mount me while we were playing horsie. That was an awkward moment, let me tell you.

Dax was in first grade when the first really big challenge came. We had fought tooth and nail to have Dax put in an inclusive classroom and things had gone smoothly for the first few months. Everyone was telling us how well Dax was doing and how hard he was trying. Then something happened that threatened all that: Dax started hating white pants. Anytime another student or teacher wore white pants Dax would become violent towards that person. He would lunge and charge, push them out of their desk or tear at their clothes.

He never seriously hurt anyone, but it was becoming a significant problem. It got to the point where Crystal and I were called to the school almost daily because Dax had gone after someone wearing white pants. The principal told us that if we couldn't get this problem under control, Dax would have to be removed from the classroom on a permanent basis.

We tried story boards. We tried timeouts. We tried corporal punishment. We tried everything. We even tried to convince Dax that there was no such thing as white pants, that the offending pants were cream colored instead of white. He didn't buy it.

Things were approaching the critical stage. Other parents had started to complain to the school about Dax's outbursts. Finally, Crystal took the gloves off. She decided the next day that she wasn't going to like whatever color pants Dax wore. She was going to go with him to school and act ugly to him all day because of the color of his pants. She was good at it too; I almost felt sorry for Dax. And you know what? It worked. Dax gained understanding by being put in the position of the people he was hurting. Crystal made Dax tell her what she could do to not be upset by the color of his pants. By having to think of ways to help Crystal, he learned to deal with his own problems. Dax's behavior improved. He had some relapses, and when he did Crystal would repeat her act the following day. Slowly but surely, the incidents slowed until Dax finally quit attacking people who wore white pants.

We've haven't had to worry about white pants in a long time. Sometimes it takes creative steps to produce the desired result. Persistence and thinking outside the box always prevail.

Between the ages of four and eight, Dax had an adventurous streak and a disturbing lack of fear (which I understand is common in autistic children). Even when he was closely supervised, it wasn't unusual to find him lying in the middle of the street, standing on the roof or jumping out of a tree. Crystal and I had to turn our house and backyard into a domestic version of Fort Knox. Ladders were kept strictly under lock and key. Buzzer alarms were placed on the front door so we would know when it was opened. We built an eight-foot-tall cinder block fence around the backyard and installed gates that couldn't be opened from inside. We even had to put an alarm on Dax's bedroom door because he liked to sneak out of his room in the early morning hours and get into mischief. Our house was like a prison. It was the only way to keep Dax out of trouble.

Dax was five when he began to intentionally injure himself during tantrums. He would run face first into a wall or jump head first off the couch. Other times he would punch himself in the face. It was horrifying just how dedicated Dax could be to hurting himself. Tantrums, at their worst, could stretch into hours. To keep Dax safe during these episodes we practiced pressure restraint, lying gently on top of him or hugging him tightly until the fit passed.

Unfortunately, this type of behavior wasn't just limited to our home. He had these tantrums at school as well. They were especially bad when they first began, since his teachers and aides were woefully unprepared to deal with his fury or his determination to self-injure. Thankfully, Dax eventually grew out of this behavior. By the time he was seven, self-injury was rare and it was gone completely by the time he was eight.

There were times Crystal and I would resent Dax for his behavior, especially if he caused a scene in a public place and embarrassed us. Dealing with the emotional backlash of these feelings was particularly rough. We'd cry over feeling that way about our son, no matter how fleeting the emotion was. But life with Dax can also be funny. The social skills of autistic children can lead to humorous and/or embarrassing moments, and Dax's skills have provided quite a few. One day we were in the grocery checkout line. A rather heavyset lady was in front of us. She accidentally backed into Dax and when she turned to apologize, Dax responded with, "You're fat." Just as blunt and loud as can be. The look she gave me could have peeled paint off walls.

Another time we were having a family dinner at Red Lobster. Dax was standing in his chair so he could better see the large aquarium across the room. The waiter had just come to take our order when Dax got an itch near his private parts, one he couldn't quite reach through his pants. Still standing in the chair, he pulled down his pants and underwear and began to scratch himself. I don't know which caused the bigger scene: Dax doing a striptease or Crystal diving across the table to pull his pants back up.

We live in an oil and mining town, so people often have the "blue collar" appearance while in convenience store lines or in the bank on payday. Lately, whenever we are next to someone who appears dirty, Dax will make a great show of sniffing the air, followed by gagging sounds and asking: "What stinks?" Subtlety is obviously not a skill he possesses.

One day at school, Dax told a girl he had a crush on, "We're going to get married and mate like killer whales." Too much Discovery Channel I guess.

One aspect of autism we found extremely difficult to deal with was the treatment we got from others. Friends and even family members distanced themselves from Dax. They were always afraid of setting off a tantrum and were scared to be around him. It really hurt when we'd leave him with his grandparents, only to have them bring him back home ten minutes later. Looks and comments from strangers hurt as well. People would glare at us when Dax was having a fit, as if to say we were horrible parents who had no control over our child. We frequently heard comments like, "If that were my son...." We'd want to scream, "You don't understand!"

Sometimes we'd feel alone, especially when friends were talking about their children performing in school plays and such. It was often easy to imagine we were the only parents in the world with a child like Dax.

But we got through it all. No matter how bad it was, we got through it.

We've had many more experiences and adventures than the handful we've shared here. It's been an exciting ten years. It has been a very rewarding ten years and, at times, a very difficult ten years. But we wouldn't trade them for the world.

Derek Neeld lives in Carlsbad, New Mexico, where he and his wife Crystal raise Dax, their ten-year-old son diagnosed with autism. They treasure each day with Dax, good or bad.

Letting Go
Arlene Palopoli

I'm certain many mothers of special needs children suffer the same fears: "What will happen when I am gone?" "Who will care for my child when I am old?" I certainly did. But as fortune would have it, we were blessed with the opportunity for Karen, our autistic daughter of 29, to move in to a group home.

As pleased as we were with this opportunity, we were concerned about how to tell Karen that she would be leaving our home to live on her own. We decided to ask our older daughter to make this the time that she would make her own move out from under Mom and Dad's roof. It worked. This move set the dialogue with Karen in motion. We talked about moving on with our lives, and the idea of our mature children no longer needing to live with Mom and Dad.

Once our older daughter moved, she became the model we would use for the concept of independent living when we talked with Karen. When took Karen to visit her sister's new apartment, we would take the opportunity to chat about her own move toward an independent life.

Karen's eventual move to the group home was definitely my most difficult experience in being her mom. After all, who could care for my "little girl" like I did? But Karen made the transition into her new "family" very smoothly, which of course made it easier on all of us.

I look back on it now and realize that while letting go is never easy, we had prepared Karen better than we could have imagined. I know that Karen's life has been enriched by her placement in that home. We, her parents who love her dearly, will always have concerns, but as I watch her vacation with her peers, go to parties and events and participate in a theater group, I see her life as a fuller and richer experience as she continues to grow. She's learned many behaviors. Perhaps that would explain how, after so many years of not hearing the words "I love you, Mom," I now hear them at the end of every phone conversation with my daughter, Karen.

Arlene Palopoli is retired and living in Florida with her husband. Karen enjoys trips to Florida and spending time with her older sister.

My Asperger Syndrome, My Travel Success

Roy A. Barnes

Travel has changed my life, despite living with Asperger syndrome. I first traveled abroad in early 1998. I joined a group tour, thinking the itinerary would fill my time with all the sightseeing and exploring I could ever hope for, all within the security of traveling with forty other people. I quickly discovered this wasn't the case: free time for exploring on our own was part of the schedule. During my time in London, I did venture out alone a few blocks from my hotel. The first time I did this, I came upon an Underground (subway) station that could take me virtually anywhere in the metropolitan area. How I wanted to go to Parliament to watch the House of Commons debate! I approached the Underground entrance, but then I suddenly froze: the steps that most others would apply in order to get from Point A to Point B were for me synonymous with being confronted with a million things to juggle simultaneously. Furthermore, I, like many people with Asperger's, take in every little bit of stimulation that my surroundings emanate. So when an environment isn't familiar, it can be too overwhelming to handle, which is what I experienced at that moment.

As a result, I restricted myself to exploring only those areas that were within walking distance of my hotel. I felt cheated: The whole city of London beckoned to me, and here I was clinging to a few blocks around Hyde Park!

We progressed southward through Europe over the next few weeks all the way to Athens, Greece. Along the way, my lack of spatial direction, also inherent in my condition, almost got me into dire straits on more than one occasion. As with London, only blocks away from my hotels in both Brussels and Innsbruck, I found myself wandering aimlessly through the night, asking myself how I would find my way back to the hotels. Only with the help of the police and at times some very conspicuous landmarks did I manage to return to the hotels, eventually. On rare occasions, I would go out with one or two people from the tour group during our free time to do some exploring off the beaten path. I relied on them to get us where we needed to be. My sense of inadequacy was only heightened by these experiences.

When I got back to the United States, I knew that something would have to change. Deep down, I knew my love for traveling and exploring was stronger than the handicaps of my condition. For almost a year and a half, the debacle of my first foreign trip haunted me. But by the autumn of 1999, I felt compelled to go back to London, vowing to travel independently on the subways and buses to all the parts of that great city no matter how scary it might seem and no matter how lost I might get.

I knew that for me to become the independent traveler that I yearned to be, I would have to take my Asperger syndrome by the horns and compensate for my shortcomings. First, I would have to study the maps extra hard before embarking overseas, using positive visualization to find my way around. Second, once abroad, I needed to find the gumption to go up to strangers and ask directions, even if it meant doing so every other block along the way. For many people with Asperger's, interacting with strangers is a challenge; we are generally not the most sociable folks.

A friend from Virginia planned to accompany me for the first part of the trip. We'd be together, but to gain confidence I'd act like I was alone while trying to figure out how to get to a certain destination. He'd only interject if I began to take a wrong turn. This technique proved to be very effective. He headed back to the States a few days before me, but I survived being alone in the city. That experience helped me on the road to traveling the world independently. A year later I would play tour guide, so to speak, as I took another friend all over London and its surrounding areas. Sometimes my sense of direction resulted in some minor inconveniences for us, but I persevered. The end result was a trip full of sightseeing successes!

Since that first fateful trip abroad, when I let my disability oppress my sense of adventure, I have traveled throughout Western Europe, China, and South Africa, mostly on my own. I've secured hotel reservations and train and bus tickets all over the world. I've challenged myself even further, journeying to Spain, Panama, and Italy: I had to be even more resourceful while visiting these countries, given that I am not fluent in Spanish or Italian. I got around fine with the aid of really detailed and user-friendly phrase books. The locals in those countries appreciated my attempts at using their language.

By 2004, I was confident enough with my experiences to submit travel articles to various publications. I've had many of them accepted. My desired to travel inspired me to confront my Asperger syndrome in a way that I wouldn't have done otherwise, which ultimately led me to a new career as a travel writer. This gave me the confidence to submit non-travel-related literary works for publication and I have had success there as well.

Having Asperger syndrome is just an obstacle. The key to overcoming obstacles is having a desire stronger than the reality of those obstacles. It is that inner quest which will lead one to find ways of overcoming the obstacles and fulfill one's dreams.

Roy A. Barnes writes from the windy plains of southeastern Wyoming. His travel-related works have been published by *Transitions Abroad*, *The Valley Advocate*, *Northwest Prime Time*, *Live Life Travel*, *C/Oasis*, and others. His works of poetry and prose have been published in *Poesia*, *Skatefic.com*, *Literary Liftoff*, *The Goblin Reader*, and *The Kid's Ark*.

Afterword

Is the Future of Autism Research to be Found in the Mirror?

Richard J. Kessler, D.O.

The puppets—one male, one female—were simple and made of wood, with flat, expressionless faces. They could make only simple, silent movements as they glided through four brief scenes to a string accompaniment. But a bent knee, a withdrawn hand, a lowered head or flailing arm produced a chorus of ooh's, aah's and giggles from the large young audience at the Brooklyn Academy of Music. From the simplest materials and the most basic of gestures, the audience had inferred a wide palette of human emotion and meaning. Amazing? Not to the legions of researchers who over the last several decades have studied age-old questions about the essence of man. They have confirmed what many have always felt in their hearts: that man is, at his core, a social creature.

Whether it be the neuroscientist studying face recognition, the anthropologist describing cooperation in early hominid hunting tactics, the child psychiatrist delineating the different types of mother-child attachment or the psychologist charting the development of empathy and "Theory of Mind" (ToM), it has become abundantly clear that the human brain is exquisitely evolved to perceive, attend to and invest in the human environment and ultimately to understand other people's emotions, behaviors and interactions. How could it not be so?

We are born with no capacity to care for ourselves and survive only because of our ability to engage caretakers in the task. What we need to know to survive, thrive and reproduce is learned in the crucible of parent/child interaction. In fact, human infants are "prewired" by evolution with the motivation and capacity to immediately establish a social relationship with their caretakers. Newborns, for example, will show a preference for the human voice (especially mothers) over other sounds and young infants the human face over other patterns.

Not surprisingly, human infants are born with a prodigious ability to imitate. Imitation of facial expressions has been demonstrated as early as 42 hours after birth. Within 2 to 3 weeks, a baby can imitate lip and tongue protrusion, mouth opening and finger movements. It is believed that these perception/action sequences help the infant to construct the earliest sense of a bodily self which unifies the infant's perceptions of others and their own felt acts. In these imitations the newborn will develop the capacity to translate between the seen behavior of others and what it is like to perform that same behavior and eventually be able "to walk in the mental shoes of the other," a capacity referred to as the "Theory of Mind" (ToM). To imitate is the beginning of knowing yourself and others and an early form of learning which eventually builds the foundation of many vital faculties: a more advanced understanding of others' emotions, actions and intentions, and of social interactions; the development of imagination; the ability to communicate first through gesture and, eventually, through language.

Yet it is only in the last decade that progress has been made in discovering the biological basis of this crucial innate mental capacity.

We owe it to a primate cousin, the macaque, and their interest in… raisins! In 1996, four researchers at the University of Parma, Italy, were studying brain activation patterns in macaques during the performance of simple motor actions like reaching for objects. One of the researchers walked into the laboratory and in full sight of one of the monkeys picked a raisin from a bowl and ate it. Surprisingly, the monkey's electrode fired and did so in the same pattern that it had in experiments when it had been picking up and eating raisins. Dr. Giacomo Rizzolatti and his colleagues traced the brain activity to the *premotor cortex*, a part of the frontal lobe of the brain responsible for the planning, selection and execution of actions. These "mirror neurons" became known as the "monkey see, monkey do neurons." They added a momentous new dimension to the concept of imitation, because the brain activation took place without the monkey doing any actual imitating. The imitation was "virtual." Could we conceptualize it as rehearsed or imagined? And do human beings have mirror neurons?

The discovery of mirror neurons set off a research revolution. Large groups of mirror neurons were discovered in humans, not just in areas of the brain associated with the observation of the gross motor behavior of others, like hand actions, but also in areas of the brain associated with facial expression, affect and speech. Numerous experiments demonstrated that human mirror neuron systems reach beyond the recognition of action to the grasping of the meaning of the action. Many neuroscientists now feel that mirror neuron systems are crucial in the development of empathy and language. In 2000, Dr. V.S. Ramachandran, an internationally renowned neurologist, declared that "mirror neurons will do for psychology what DNA did for biology: they will provide a unifying framework and help explain a host of mental abilities that have hitherto remained mysterious and inaccessible to experiments." Whether that will prove to be true or not, it seems clear that human beings are born with brains that silently and automatically record the actions and interactions of others and therefore prepare them for the lifelong, life saving and life affirming activities of human relationships.

Dr. Ramachandran and many others quickly realized that mirror neuron dysfunctions could be connected to autism. Dr. Hugo Theoret of the University of Montreal has stated "If you imagine the behavioral and social deficits that would come from a failure of the mirror neuron system, you would imagine a pathology just like autism." Certainly, many of the earliest signs of autism, like the absence of joint attention behaviors and reciprocal play, strongly resonate with the idea of difficulties in establishing an inner "conversation" with another's mind in your mind. Therefore, this system seems to represent the template for the development of a Theory of Mind: the ability to understand the intentions and emotions of others, which is thought to be deficient or even absent in autism. In fact, even before the discovery of mirror neurons it had pretty much been established that children with autism had an "imitative deficit." Additionally, some have suggested that the development of stereotyped movements, rituals and the narrow interests of the autistic individual could be traced to miscarried or poorly regulated imitation.

But is there any direct evidence that autistic individuals have defective mirror neuron systems? The evidence seems to be mounting that they do. Dr. Ramachandran provided the first bit of evidence. In 2005, he recorded EEGs, or the brain wave patterns, of high functioning autistic individuals and control subjects while they watched videos of their own hands and other people's hands moving. In normal brain functioning, the *mu rhythm*, a reflection of the mirror neuron system, should be suppressed when observing one's own or another's activity. In the autistic individuals, however, the suppression occurred only in response to viewing their own activity and not the activity of others. In 2007, using a similar EEG methodology, researchers lead by Dr. Rafael Bernier at the University of Washington demonstrated that decreased mu rhythm attenuation was correlated with diminished imitation skills in autistic individuals.

In 2006, in an experiment performed at UCLA by Dr. Mirella Dapretto and her team, children with autism underwent *magnetic resonance imaging* brain scans while imitating and observing emotional expressions (anger, fear, sadness, happiness). It was found that the greater the social deficit suffered by the child, the less activity in a key part of the mirror neuron system was observed. The autistic children also showed reduced activity in a part of the brain associated with emotions, the *limbic system*, which may explain why they could imitate facial expressions but not understand the corresponding emotional state. Using a different methodology, in 2005 a Boston University research group led by Dr. Helen Tager-Flusberg found decreases in cerebral cortex thickness in autistic adults in areas belonging to the mirror neuron system as well as areas important to emotional and social cognition. These areas of cortical thinning correlated with the severity of the symptoms displayed by the autistic adult. Later, she also found diminished activity in mirror neuron systems in autistic adults watching the hand movements of others. And finally, a team from Aberdeen University headed by Dr. Justin Williams has demonstrated that the most marked differences in mirror neuron functioning in adolescent autistic boys are to be found in an area of the brain associated with ToM functioning.

Although this research appears quite promising, it is still quite early in the game. The next few years should bear work of greater depth and breadth and intersection with other areas of exploration. At the Seaver Center at Mt. Sinai Medical Center in New York City, a possible connection between *oxytocin*, a hormone that plays a crucial role in mother/child bonding and mirror neuron functioning, is under investigation. Experiments have demonstrated that this hormone, which has been shown to facilitate the processing of social information, when delivered in a nasal spray, improves subjects' performance on tasks that measure ToM abilities.

It is unlikely that a dysfunctional mirror neuron system will explain all the symptoms of autism, nor do we have as yet any clear explanation of how the system becomes dysfunctional in the first place. Moreover, the autism spectrum is indeed quite wide. After all, dozens of different, rare genetic mutations have been found to be associated with the disorders on the spectrum. Yet this work with the mirror neuron system does seem to resonate across many disciplines, confirming decades of "hunches," and also seems to corroborate many strategies used for early intervention in the areas of education and socialization. Hopefully, this research will soon begin to offer refinements of these techniques as well as new methodologies.

One thing is certain: given the central role of social relatedness in human nature, future research in autism will not just provide more clues to its origins, treatment and prevention but also a window into discovery of the means by which our species evolved. The more we access the world of autistic individuals the more we will learn about ours.

Dr. Richard J. Kessler is the Medical Director of Adults and Children with Learning and Developmental Disabilities, an organization serving over 3,000 developmentally disabled children and adults throughout Long Island, New York. He is a board-certified psychiatrist, a Distinguished Fellow of the American Psychiatric Association, Assistant Clinical Professor at Albert Einstein College of Medicine, and a member of the faculty at the Psychoanalytic Institute at New York University Medical Center.

Resentences

On the following pages you will find information on some of the foremost organizations in the country focused on autism research, treatment, and support. All of these and many, many more may be found within the Resources Section of The Healing Project's website at www.thehealingproject.org.

National Organizations and General Resources

Autism Speaks
2 Park Avenue, 11th Floor
New York, NY 10016
Phone: (212) 252-8584
Fax: (212) 252-8676
http://www.autismspeaks.org/
contactus@autismspeaks.org

Dedicated to funding global biomedical research into the causes, prevention, treatments, and cure for autism; to raising public awareness about autism and its effects on individuals, families, and society; and to bringing hope to all who deal with the hardships of this disorder.

Autism Society of America
7910 Woodmont Avenue, Suite 300
Bethesda, MD 20814-3067
Phone: (301) 657-0881 or (800) 3AUTISM (800-328-8476)
http://www.autism-society.org/site/PageServer

Autism Research Institute
4182 Adams Avenue
San Diego, CA 92116
Autism Resource Call Center: (866) 366-3361
fax: (619) 563-6840
http://www.autism.com/index.htm

ARI was founded in 1967 to conduct and foster scientific research designed to improve the methods of diagnosing, treating, and preventing autism, and to disseminate research findings to parents and others seeking help. The ARI data bank, the world's largest, contains over 40,000 detailed case histories of autistic children from over 60 countries.

National Autism Association
1330 W. Schatz Lane
Nixa, MO 65714
Phone: (877) NAPA-AUTISM (877-622-2884)
http://www.nationalautismassociation.org/
naa@nationalautism.org

The mission of the National Autism Association is to educate and empower families affected by autism and other neurological disorders, while advocating on behalf of those who cannot fight for their own rights.

Autism Today
United States Office:
Exceptional Resources, Inc.
1425 Broadway #444
Seattle, WA 98122
Phone: (866) 9AUTISM (866-928-8476)

Canadian Office:
Autism Today Education Corporation
2016 Sherwood Drive, Suite 3

Sherwood Park, Alberta, Canada T8A 3X3
Phone: (780) 482-1555
Fax: (780) 452-1098
http://www.autismtoday.com/index.asp

Autism Today seeks to simplify the information gathering and evaluating process for families dealing with autism spectrum disorders.

National Institute of Child Health and Human Development
P.O. Box 3006
Rockville, MD 20847
Phone: (800) 370-2943
TTY: (888) 320-6942
Fax: (301) 984-1473
http://www.nichd.nih.gov/
NICHDInformationResourceCenter@mail.nih.gov

The NICHD, established by Congress in 1962, conducts and supports research on topics related to the health of children, adults, families, and populations.

Center for Autism and Related Disorders
CARD Corporate Headquarters
19019 Ventura Boulevard, Suite 300
Tarzana, CA 91356
Phone: (818) 345-2345
Fax: (818) 758-8015
http://www.centerforautism.com/
info@centerforautism.com

Center for Autism and Related Disorders, Inc. (CARD) has several offices around the world and is among the world's largest and most experienced organizations effectively treating children with autism and related disorders.

Kennedy Kreiger Institute
707 North Broadway
Baltimore, MD 21205
Phone: (443) 923-9200 or (800) 873-3377
http://www.kennedykrieger.org/
info@kennedykrieger.org.

Kennedy Krieger Institute is an internationally recognized facility dedicated to improving the lives of children and adolescents with pediatric developmental disabilities through patient care, special education, research, and professional training.

Centers for Disease Control and Prevention Autism Information Center
1600 Clifton Road
Atlanta, GA 30333
Phone: (404) 639-3534 or (800) 311-3435
http://www.cdc.gov/ncbddd/autism/

CDC's mission is to promote health and quality of life by preventing and controlling disease, injury, and disability.

American Academy of Pediatrics
141 Northwest Point Boulevard
Elk Grove Village, IL 60007
Phone: (847) 434-4000
Fax: (847) 434-8000
http://www.aap.org/

The American Academy of Pediatrics is an organization of 60,000 pediatricians committed to the attainment of optimal physical, mental, and social health and well-being for all infants, children, adolescents, and young adults.

Southwest Autism Research & Resource Center (SARRC)
Campus for Exceptional Children
300 N. 18th Street
Phoenix, AZ 85006-4103
Phone: (602) 340-8717
Fax: (602) 340-8720
http://www.autismcenter.org/
sarrc@autismcenter.org

SARRC models and promotes best practices that enhance the quality of life for children and adults with autism spectrum disorders, empowers children, families, and professionals with information and training, and advances discoveries that will ultimately lead to a cure.

National Institute of Neurological Disorders and Stroke
NIH Neurological Institute
P.O. Box 5801
Bethesda, MD 20824
Phone: (800) 352-9424 or (301) 496-5751
TTY: (301) 468-5981
http://www.ninds.nih.gov/

The National Institute of Neurological Disorders and Stroke (NINDS) conducts and supports research on brain and nervous system disorders. Created by Congress in 1950, NINDS is one of the more than two dozen research institutes and centers that comprise the National Institutes of Health (NIH).

Yale Child Study Center Autism/PDD Clinic
Yale Child Study Center
230 South Frontage Road
P.O. Box 207900
New Haven, CT 06520-7900
Fax: (203) 737-4197
http://info.med.yale.edu/chldstdy/autism/

The Yale Developmental Disabilities Clinic offers comprehensive, multidisciplinary evaluations for children with social disabilities, usually focusing on the issues of diagnosis and intervention.

**National Dissemination Center for Children
with Disabilities (NICHCY)**
P.O. Box 1492
Washington, DC 20013
Phone: (800) 695-0285
Fax: (202) 884-8441
http://www.nichcy.org/
nichcy@aed.org

A central source of information on: disabilities in infants, toddlers, children, and youth; IDEA, which is the law authorizing special education; No Child Left Behind (as it relates to children with disabilities); and research-based information on effective educational practices.

The Center for Human Policy
Syracuse University, School of Education
805 South Crouse Avenue
Syracuse, NY 13244-2280
http://thechp.syr.edu//
razubal@syr.edu

The Center on Human Policy (CHP) is a Syracuse University–based policy, research, and advocacy organization involved in the national movement to insure the rights of people with disabilities. Since its founding, the Center has been involved in the study and promotion of open settings (inclusive community opportunities) for people with disabilities.

Waisman Center
University of Wisconsin-Madison
1500 Highland Avenue

Madison, WI 53705-2280
http://www.familyvillage.wisc.edu/
familyvillage@waisman.wisc.edu

A global community that integrates information, resources, and communication opportunities on the Internet for persons with cognitive and other disabilities, for their families, and for those who provide them services and support.

TASH (disability advocacy group)
1025 Vermont Avenue NW, 7th Floor
Washington, DC 20005
Phone: (202) 263-5600
Fax: (202) 637-0138
http://www.tash.org/index.html

TASH is an international membership association leading the way to inclusive communities through research, education, and advocacy. TASH members are people with disabilities, family members, fellow citizens, advocates, and professionals working together to create change and build capacity so that all people, no matter their perceived level of disability, are included in all aspects of society.

Kids Together, Inc.
P.O. Box 574
Quakertown, PA 18954
http://www.kidstogether.org/
staff@kidstogether.org

Its mission is to promote inclusive communities where all people belong.

LD OnLine: Learning Disabilities Resources
WETA Public Television
2775 S. Quincy Street
Arlington, VA 22206

Fax: (703) 998-2060
http://www.ldonline.org/
http://www.ldonline.org/sitecontact

LD OnLine.org is the world's leading website on learning disabilities and ADHD, serving more than 250,000 parents, teachers,
and other professionals each month.

The Boulevard
jjMarketing, Inc.
1205 Savoy Street, Suite 101
San Diego, CA 92107
Phone: (619) 222-8735
Fax: (619) 226-2675
http://www.blvd.com/

A resource directory of products and services for the physically
challenged, elderly, caregivers, and healthcare professionals.

Council for Exceptional Children
Ballston Plaza Two
1110 North Glebe Road, Suite 300
Arlington, VA 22201-5704
Phone: (800) 224-6830
http://www.cec.sped.org//AM/Template.cfm?Section=Home

Dedicated to improving educational outcomes for individuals
with exceptionalities, students with disabilities, and/or the gifted,
CEC advocates for appropriate governmental policies, sets professional standards, provides continual professional development,
advocates for newly and historically underserved individuals with
exceptionalities, and helps professionals obtain conditions and
resources necessary for effective professional practice.

Association for Persons in Supported Employment
1627 Monument Avenue
Richmond, VA 23220
Phone: (804) 278-9187
Fax: (804) 278-9377
http://www.apse.org/
apse@apse.org

Supported employment (SE) enables people with disabilities who have not been successfully employed to work and contribute to society. SE focuses on a person's abilities and provides the supports the individual needs to be successful on a long-term basis.

Federation for Children with Special Needs
1135 Tremont Street, Suite 420
Boston, MA 02120
Phone: (617) 236-7210 or (800) 331-0688 (in MA)
Fax: (617) 572-2094
http://fcsn.org/index.php
fcsninfo@fcsn.org

The Federation operates a Parent Center in Massachusetts which offers a variety of services to parents, parent groups, and others who are concerned with children with special needs.

National Association on Disability
910 Sixteenth Street, NW, Suite 600
Washington, DC 20006
Phone: (202) 293-5960
Fax: (202) 293-7999
TTY: (202) 293-5968
http://www.nod.org/
ability@nod.org

The mission of the National Organization on Disability (NOD) is to expand the participation and contribution of America's 54 million men, women, and children with disabilities in all aspects of life.

National Rehabilitation Information Center (NARIC)

8201 Corporate Drive, Suite 600
Landover, MD 20785
Phone: (800) 346-2742 or (301) 459-5900
http://www.naric.com/
naricinfo@heitechservices.com

Offers disability- and rehabilitation-oriented information organized in a variety of formats.

RESNA

1700 N. Moore Street, Suite 1540
Arlington, VA 22209-1903
Phone: (703) 524-6686
Fax: (703) 524-6630
www.resna.org
info@resna.org

The mission of RESNA is to improve the potential of people with disabilities to achieve their goals through the use of technology. It promotes research, development, education, advocacy, and provision of technology; and supports the people engaged in these activities.

Access to Respite Care and Help (ARCH)

800 Eastown Drive, Suite 105
Chapel Hill, NC 27514
Phone: (919) 490-5577
Fax: (919) 490-4905
http://www.chtop.com/

ARCH develops, demonstrates, and delivers programs and strategies that will enhance the lives of children, youth, and families. Of principal concern to project staff are families in poverty, families caring for the elderly, children with disabilities or chronic illness, and children at risk of abuse and neglect.

Associaton of University Centers on Disabilities
1010 Wayne Avenue, Suite 920
Silver Spring, MD 20910
Phone: (301) 588-8252
Fax: (301) 588-2842
http://www.aucd.org/template/index.cfm

AUCD's mission is to advance policy and practice for and with people with developmental and other disabilities, their families and their communities by supporting our members in research, education, and service activities.

Administration for Families and Children:
Administration on Developmental Disabilities
370 L'Enfant Promenade, SW
Washington, DC 20201
http://www.acf.dhhs.gov/acf_contact_us.html
http://www.acf.dhhs.gov/programs/add/

The Administration on Developmental Disabilities (ADD) is the U.S. government organization responsible for implementation of the Developmental Disabilities Assistance and Bill of Rights Act of 2000, known as the ADD Act. ADD, its staff and programs, are part of the Administration for Children and Families of the U.S. Department of Health and Human Services.

Resources on Education/Special Education

National Early Childhood Technical Assistance System
Campus Box 8040, UNC-CH
Chapel Hill, NC 27599-8040
Phone: (919) 962-2001
TDD: (919) 843-3269
Fax: (919) 966-7463
http://www.nectas.unc.edu/
nectac@unc.edu

Web clearinghouse of information on early childhood development.

U.S. Department of Education

400 Maryland Avenue, SW
Washington, DC 20202
Phone: (800) USA-LEARN (800-872-5327)
TTY: (800) 437-0833
Fax: (202) 401-0689
http://www.ed.gov/index.jhtml

Promotes improvements in the quality and usefulness of education through Federally supported research, evaluation, and sharing of information.

Other Products and Services

Different Roads to Learning

37 East 18th Street, 10th Floor
New York, NY 10003
Phone: (800) 853-1057
Fax: (800) 317-9146
http://www.difflearn.com/
info@difflearn.com

Over 250 products for children with autism, including books, flashcards, and videos, along with other materials critical to Applied Behavior Analysis and Verbal Behavior programs.

Laureate Learning Systems

110 East Spring Street
Winooski, VT 05404-1898
Phone: (800) 562-6801 or (802) 655-4755
Fax: (802) 655-4757
http://www.laureatelearning.net/professionals602/

Dedicated to publishing innovative software of the highest quality, specifically designed to improve the lives of children and adults with special needs. Laureate's multimedia programs combine superior instructional design with digital speech, engaging graphics, and amusing animation.

James Stanfield Publishing Company
Drawer: WEB
P.O. Box 41058
Santa Barbara, CA 93140
Phone: (800) 421-6534
Fax: (805) 897-1187
http://www.stanfield.com/
orderdesk@stanfield.com

The company offers a library of educational materials in the areas of conflict management for the general school population and for students with cognitive challenges.

Crestwood Company: Communication Aids for Children and Adults
P.O. Box 090107
Milwaukee, WI 53209-0107
Phone: (414) 352-5678
Fax: (414) 352-5679
http://www.communicationaids.com/
crestcomm@aol.com

Crestwood offers communication devices to help children and adults express their thoughts and needs.

Dimensions
12545 Orange Drive, Suite 502
Davie, Florida 33330
Phone: (954) 236-9415
Fax: (954) 236-9405
http://www.dimensionsspeech.com/
info@dimensionstherapycenter.com

Provides state-of-the-art therapy services in a motivating and structured format.

Attention Control Systems
650 Castro Street, Suite 120, PMB 197
Mountain View, CA 94041
Phone: (650) 494-2002
Fax: (650) 493-2002
www.brainaid.com
info@brainaid.com

Offers computerized planning for people with cognitive disorders.

The Association for the Neurologically Disabled of Canada
The A.N.D Centre
59 Clement Road
Etobicoke, Ontario
Canada M9R 1Y5
Phone: (416) 244-1992 / (800) 561-1497
Fax: (416) 244-4099
www.and.ca
info@and.ca

A.N.D. Canada is a nonprofit charitable organization dedicated to providing functional rehabilitation programs to individuals with neurological disabilities. Its unique home-based, non-institutionalized rehabilitation program attempts to stimulate the brain's ability to develop despite injury or inadequate development.

SNCARC: South Norfolk County
Association for Retarded Citizens
South Norfolk County Arc
789 Clapboardtree Street
Westwood, MA 02090
Phone: (781) 762-4001
Fax: (781) 461-5950
http://www.sncarc.org/
dwood@sncarc.org

Advocates for and provides supports and services to people disabled by mental retardation and other developmental disabilities, and to their families.

Suffolk AHRC: Suffolk County, New York chapter of AHRC
2900 Veterans Memorial Highway
Bohemia, NY 11716
Phone: (631) 585-0100
http://www.ahrcsuffolk.org/

Provides programs and services for over 2,500 men, women, and children with developmental disabilities.

Institutes for Human Potential
8801 Stenton Avenue
Wyndmoor, PA 19038
Phone: (215) 233-2050
Fax: (215) 233-9312
http://www.iahp.org
institutes@iahp.org

A nonprofit educational organization that serves children by introducing parents to the field of early child development. Parents learn how to enhance the development of their children physically, intellectually, and socially in a joyous and sensible way.

National Academy for Child Development
549 25th Street
Ogden, UT 84401-2422
Phone: (801) 621-8606
Fax: (801) 621-8389
http://www.nacd.org/

NACD provides neurodevelopmental evaluations and individualized programs for children and adults, updated on a quarterly basis.

Information on Attention Deficit Disorder

ADDA
15000 Commerce Parkway, Suite C
Mount Laurel, NJ 08054
Phone: (856) 439-9099, (856) 439-0525
http://www.add.org/
adda@ahint.com

The Attention Deficit Disorder Association provides information, resources, and networking to adults with AD/HD and to the professionals who work with them.

Information on Angelman Syndrome

Angelman Syndrome Foundation
P.O. Box 31700
Omaha, NE 68131-0700
Phone: (877) CSA-4CSA
Fax: (402) 558-1347
http://www.angelman.org/

ASF's mission is to advance the awareness and treatment of Angelman syndrome through education and information, research, and support for individuals with Angelman syndrome, their families, and other concerned parties.

Information on Celiac Disease

Celiac Sprue Association/United States of America
P.O. Box 31700
Omaha, NE 68131-0700
Phone: (877) CSA-4CSA
Fax: (402) 558-1347
http://www.csaceliacs.org/
celiacs@csaceliacs.org

Celiac Sprue Association/United States of America, Inc. (CSA/USA, Inc.) is a member-based nonprofit organization dedicated to helping individuals with celiac disease and dermatitis herpetiformis worldwide through education, research, and support.

Information on Epilepsy

Epilepsy Foundation of America

8301 Professional Place
Landover, MD 20785
Phone: (800) 332-1000
http://www.epilepsyfoundation.org/

The Epilepsy Foundation is the national voluntary agency solely dedicated to the welfare of the over 3 million people with epilepsy in the U.S. and their families. The organization works to ensure that people with seizures are able to participate in all life experiences; and to prevent, control, and cure epilepsy through research, education, advocacy, and services.

Information on Hyperlexia and Semantic Pragmatic Disorder

American Hyperlexia Association

479 Spring Road
Elmhurst, IL 60126
Phone: (630) 415-2212
Fax: (630) 530-5909
http://www.hyperlexia.org/
info@hyperlexia.org

The American Hyperlexia Association is dedicated to the advancement of the education and general welfare of children with hyperlexia. It advocates and encourages research related to hyperlexia and seeks to assist families of children with hyperlexia in accessing appropriate services.

Information on Learning Disabilities

Learning Disabilities Association of America (LDA)
4156 Library Road
Pittsburgh, PA 15234-1349
Phone: (412) 341-1515
Fax: (412) 344-0224
http://www.ldanatl.org/

A national organization that serves tens of thousands of members with learning disabilities, their families, and the professionals who work with them.

Information on Fragile X Syndrome

FRAXA / Fragile-X Syndrome
45 Pleasant Street
Newburyport, MA 01950
Phone: (978) 462-1866
http://www.fraxa.org/

FRAXA's mission is to accelerate progress toward effective treatments and ultimately a cure for Fragile X by directly funding the most promising research.

Information on PDD

Autism/PDD Resources Network
14271 Jeffrey #3
Irvine, CA 92620
http://www.autism-pdd.net/

Autism-PDD.Net is an information and resource site for parents of children and caregivers coping with autism.

Information on Music Therapy

American Music Therapy Association, Inc.
8455 Colesville Road, Suite 1000
Silver Spring, MD 20910
Phone: (301) 589-3300
Fax: (301) 589-5175
http://www.musictherapy.org/
info@musictherapy.org

The American Music Therapy Association advances public awareness of the benefits of music therapy and increase access to quality music therapy services in a rapidly changing world.

Music Therapy Association of British Columbia
2055 Purcell Way
North Vancouver, BC
V7J 3H5
Phone: (604) 924-0046
Fax: (604) 983-7559
http://www.mtabc.com/
info@mtabc.com